EAT YOUR ASS OFF ...literally!

With Dr. Emerson's 16/21 Diet Solution

Lose Weight & Keep It Off
Lower Cholesterol
Increase Your Energy
& Live a Healthier Life

Mark D. Emerson, DC, CCSP

Emerson, Mark, 1966–

Eat Your Ass Off…Literally: with Dr. Emerson's 16/21 Diet Solution.
The Easy, Fool Proof Method To Lose Weight & Keep It Off, Lower Cholesterol, Increase Your Energy & Live a Healthier Life.

This book is intended to be informational and should not be considered a substitute for advice from a medical professional. The reader should consult a medical professional before beginning any diet or exercise regime and before taking any dietary supplements or other medications. The author expressly disclaim responsibility for any adverse effects arising from the use or application of the information contained in this book.

For informational purposes only, I have mentioned and listed companies, brand names, individuals, multiple books and websites. I believe the information would be helpful to readers, but to my knowledge, I have no connections to any of the companies, brand names, or products with the exception of DocEmerson Co., which is the company I founded. DocEmerson, DocEmerson's Perfect Living Series, and The 16/21 Diet Solution are trademarks and service marks of DocEmerson Co. www.docemerson.com.

ISBN 978-0-615-33722-7

Published by: DocEmerson Co., Tampa, Florida 33616

Dedications

This book is dedicated to:

My Children: **Gregory, Derek, Miles and Gabriela;**

You have given my life the most important purpose. Thank you for your unconditional love and the wisdom that children provide for parents to learn and grow. I love you with all my heart and soul. Semper Fidelis!

My mother, **Mert**, for always having the strength to continue on.

My sister **Beverly**, for your unconditional love and support.

My sister **Rhonda**, for giving my childhood love and room to dream.

My sister **Sheree**, for enduring the inhumane cruelty that overweight children and adults suffer by very mean people. Your plight has been a major stimulus in my desire to help people.

Kathy, the noblest and most principled of assistants. You have always been there as a support, source of strength and reality checker. Thank you for being the glue that held me together at the toughest of times and kicking me in the backside when needed. This work could not have been completed without your support.

Dr. Michael Klaper for your inspiration, friendship, advice and support. Your dedicated work in the world of nutritional science is invaluable to all mankind.

In Loving Memory: **Dr. Phillip Albert Cernius** for always going beyond the call of duty. This world is not the same without you, but I know the next one is grateful for your arrival. Your loving brother, Odie.

Table of Contents

Foreword

One of the most difficult issues you may face in your life is when your health is compromised or challenged. Whether you want to lose weight, reduce your blood pressure or cholesterol, or heal from a major illness, there is no greater daunting task.

Our health status is quintessentially a snap shot of how we eat. If we eat well, our health is generally good. Conversely, if we eat junk, our health is junk. Throughout my many years as a healthcare provider, I have found that nearly everything that affects our health, especially **weight** and **energy** issues, stem from what we are doing to ourselves through our daily eating choices. Eating is a necessary and colossal component to our existence. Without it, we do not thrive, grow, heal and prosper. However, eating poorly is the **main** cause of sickness and disease.

This book is a realistic, non-BS approach to help you understand how to improve your health and life. This book may push your comfort zone regarding your current eating choices. There are long standing misconceptions about proper diet, foods and nutritional requirements that perpetuate the poor health that plagues society. This book will show you how eating healthier is easy, wonderful and the benefits come quickly. You will also discover that you can still be **you**. It is about how you were designed by nature, not disconnecting you from who you are as a person. There are no guilt trips or shame in my system. My goal is to bring to light the miraculous healing ability you have within to help you live a healthier, happy life.

If you are ready to make solid, workable changes to improve your life and health, then this will be as easy as 1-2-3. So go ahead, Eat your ass off, literally and **enjoy**!

A Healthy Understanding from Early On

I have been a natural healthcare practitioner since 1990. The integration of proper nutrition has always been a cornerstone of my treatment philosophy in helping patients improve their health.

Prior to my formal training, my initial education and understanding of nutrition actually started to blossom in my childhood. I grew up in Northern California in the 1960's and 70's during a time in which progressive thought toward spirituality and healthy living exploded. Though I was among the younger generation of the time, as I was born in 1966, my oldest sister was graduating high school the same week I was making my intro into this world. My two older sisters and two brothers in-law are 18 and 16 years older than me. It was their "flower children" generation that had a wonderful and lasting shaping of my holistic education.

I found it captivating to soak in the "hippie" thought process towards **natural living** and eating a diet that was back to nature and away from chemical processing. I innocently and luckily took the essence of their natural living ideas, which actually echoed many of our most profound thinkers of human history from Plato to Gandhi to Ben Franklin to even Jesus. These historical heroes all knew the importance of healthy eating. The late 60's and early 70's was the time when our country bathed in philosophical expansion and the infinite possibilities to find peace, harmony and health.

As I continued my pursuit of understanding healing and human physiology, I discovered there were many published reports by respected physicians in the early 1900's documenting the importance of proper nutrition to acheive good health. These early reports showed a clinical intervention using a diet rich in whole grains, vegetables and fruits to treat the sick and keep the healthy healthy, with wonderful results. If you think about it, most all of the dangerous conditions of the past, such as scurvy, beriberi and rickets were actually nutrient deficiencies. Once given the proper nutrients, the diseases were resolved.

This is true for most health problems. Unfortunately, as time went **on big business** got in the way of healthy logic and we now live in a country where most of our sickness is caused by a poor diet once again. A diet lacking in human nutritional needs.

Early in my practice, I realized it is extremely difficult for people to make changes in their lives, especially with eating habits. That is what stimulated me to design a dietary system that is highly nutritious, great tasting and does not require you to make drastic changes for you to experience the positive benefits.

I owe a world of gratitude for my comprehensive knowledge of the healing arts to my older sisters and to their generation. For it is their generation, who started as the "flower children" and now are the "baby boomers" that stimulated my calling as a healer and health expert.

It is my hope that people of all ages will take the wisdom that has been handed down to me and enhanced with my clinical experience to heart. It is **possible** to truly enjoy a healthy and healing diet and live in **good health**.

Many lifestyle changes require big changes to our mind-set. Many of us, myself included, are set in our ways a bit. I designed **The 16/21 Diet Solution** to offer people real world solutions to healthier eating because I do not think you need to turn your world upside down to get great results.

Keep the big picture! ☺

Fast Forward to the Present

Our society is plagued with so many illnesses and syndromes that most health experts agree that a poor diet is the main contributor to poor health. A poor diet has been shown to be a direct link to conditions such as:

- **Heart Disease (the #1 killer in the US)**
- **Obesity or Overweight Problems**
- **High Blood Pressure**
- **Diabetes**
- **Many Cancers**
- **Chronic Fatigue**
- **Depression/Anxiety**
- **Attention Deficit Disorder**

The most current medical research is showing the negative effects of **chronic inflammation**, as it appears to be a catalyst for all the major diseases. Not surprisingly, chronic inflammation appears to be caused and perpetuated by a poor diet as well.

Additionally, **weight loss** and **anti-aging** solutions continue to dominate the want list of people everywhere. Poor health has affected so many people, that suffering from a disease or a condition has become accepted as "normal" aspects of modern day living or aging.

However, these conditions are not normal. These conditions are pathogenic and sadly, in most cases, self-inflicted. The bright side: they are correctable and preventable. A proper diet can even reverse disease, as Dr. Dean Ornish proved with cardiovascular patients. I am convinced, based upon my years of clinical experience, that a proper diet can restore your health from most conditions.

It is important to understand that, due to our poor dietary habits, we are losing our most precious natural resource. That precious natural resource is **good health** and it is falling like bad stocks.

Sadly, our declining health has even reached down to the most innocent of souls, our children. Children, as young as 5 years old, are now clinically obese. Many lifestyle choices can be blamed, from video games, to television, to both parents working, but blaming does not correct anything.

The root of the problem that is affecting your health more than any other variable is **what** you are eating on a daily basis. That is the problem.

I believe many people understand that a poor diet is causing their health problems. I also believe many people understand the idea;

"You are what you eat."

This profound age-old adage tells the story of the health status of every man, woman and child.

However, as a population, we are so confused as to which guru fad "diet" to follow next, that eating healthy has become more of a chore than applicable wisdom, and the "poor health" cycle is never fixed.

As I read many of the "diet" book strategies, I see the problem. Many are too extreme, instructing you to polarize to a particular dogma with too restrictive food choices. Other diets align too closely to the Standard American Diet (SAD) and perpetuate the lack of nutrients your body needs for health. The *Atkins Diet* is a prime example of an unsound "diet." Many "diet plans" are just gimmicks, no different from the "work from home 3 hours a week and make $8K per month." Yeah right, whatever! So the confusion continues and it is very frustrating.

However, the importance of eating better is talked about everywhere. Even from the most reputable health organizations. For example:

> **The World Health Organization states:**
> *"An unhealthy diet is one of the major risk factors for a range of chronic diseases, including cardiovascular diseases, cancer, diabetes and other conditions linked to obesity. Specific recommendations for a healthy diet include: cutting down on salt, sugar and fat; eating more fruit, vegetables, nuts and grains; and substituting unsaturated vegetable oils for saturated animal fats"*

It is true, when you see the list of diseases that are killing us, the top 5 are directly related to what we are eating. No mystery at all. The mystery for me was to design a system that actually works and is user friendly enough for people to stick to. This is why I created a successful diet protocol by using a real-world approach.

My 16/21 Diet Solution is an honest, realistic approach to healthy eating. It offers you permanent dietary solutions that can be applied throughout your entire life. It is designed to correct your body's ability to function better and improve your health.

It is clinically designed and backed by nutritional science. I call it a dietary solution because that is what it is. It is not a fad "diet" that you will end up hating due to roller coaster results; it is a dietary system that gives you the **results** you want. I am sure you have heard the saying:

> *"The definition of insanity is doing the same thing over and over and expecting different results."*

That's what "dieting" is!!

No matter what your health goal is, you must get healthier to improve your life. And your can only get healthier by eating better. If you are ready to lose unwanted, unhealthy pounds, lower your cholesterol and blood pressure, reverse or prevent heart disease, and increase your level of health without toxic drugs or fad diets, then The 16/21 Diet Solution is for you.

If you follow the advice within The 16/21 Diet Solution, you'll lose the unhealthy weight for the last time, never count calories, and eat as much as you desire. The benefits are not only for those who are overweight. They are for anyone who wants to protect their most precious resource...their health.

Throughout the book, I will refer to my healthy eating design as: The 16/21 Solution, The 16/21 Diet Solution, 16/21 or The Solution. It doesn't matter to me what you want to call it. What matters is that you apply the simple, easy to follow and great tasting way to better health. The word "diet" has been used for nearly everything in marketing. However, if you look up the origin of the word, "**diet**" means "a way of life."

Profoundly, it means just that. If you eat unhealthy, your "way of life" is unhealthy; and if you eat well and healthy, you live well and healthy.

The Keys to Success:

1. **Achieving better health is a process and a path. Therefore, have a little patience and allow yourself forgiveness.**
2. **Expect to make bad choices and slip-ups and don't sweat it when you do. You will blow it; we all do, but don't worry. Just keep on the path.**
3. **Allow yourself time to acclimate to the new tastes and new flavors of eating better. Don't expect everything to taste like the junk you have been eating. That is what got you into a world of hurt to start with. You will discover, foods that are healing taste great.**
4. **Apply what you learn in this book and in a short time, you will see the amazing results of good health.**

By applying my easy-to-follow principles, you will see dramatic, positive results within 30 days. Stick with it and the results and benefits will be life-long. You will find that you will not be "missing" stuff that you think you cannot live without. My diet design is to help you eat your way to good health. If you desire to be healthier, this book will get you there.

CHAPTER 1

How Your Body Works and Why You Are Crashing and Burnin'

As I stated, it is commonly understood that poor eating habits create poor health. Therefore, it is essential to know what to eat. But before anyone sets out to improve their health, lose weight, reach fitness goals or slow the aging process, it is imperative to understand, even in simple terms, **how your body works**. If you have this basic, helpful knowledge you can have great results.

Every single day, your body works to keep you healthy and strong. It is designed to **elevate your health** because it is programmed from conception to do so. You literally live in the most miraculous invention possible. If you could patent the design and all the abilities the human mind and body are capable of into an income stream, your net worth would make Bill Gates' financial statement look like a welfare check. That is how invaluable your body systems are to your **quality of life**.

Your body is so well-designed that it actually works effectively despite what you do to it. Every cell of your body works in harmony with all the other cells to orchestrate your living being. Your body is a very intrinsic and complex design, and it works perfectly without you needing to comprehend all that is going on.

This is the internal wisdom of your body and it operates continually, taking care of you at all times; always assessing, repairing, growing, and protecting. Your body is designed to work like a fine-tuned orchestra. Nature blessed you with an outstanding hard drive and a flawless operating system. It works so well, that many of us can continue to live each day with ongoing chronic conditions or problems. However, when you are living with problematic conditions, your body is forced into orchestrating damage control and survival mode, more than good health or well-being.

Imagine if your body was working at an elevated level of performance all the time. Imagine the quality of life and health you would have if you were feeling how you should be. Living well, feeling healthy, strong and energetic.

The secret to having the good health you want is to know what to feed your body. Feed your body correctly and your body will take care of you. It is the deal of the millennium. It is a win-win situation for you. If you keep your end of the bargain, your body rewards you by elevating, regaining and restoring your health, regardless of what is ailing you. Aliments become short-term inconveniences instead of full-time conditions.

Here is something to remember: For your body to run all of the complex processes of repair, maintenance, growth, detoxification, and **immunity**, your body requires **energy**! How do we get this energy?

1. **Energy comes from one fuel source.**
2. **That fuel source is food.**
3. **Period!**

Fortunately, we lucked out. We live on a planet that provides us with all the **food** we need, grown right here, everyday all around the world. But to our own demise, we have also invented lots and lots of other little things that we eat that are **not food**, nor are they even close to being good for us.

Let me show you in a nutshell what keeps you alive, thriving and living in the prosperity of good health.

By nature's design, your body takes in **energy via food** and breaks it down. This energy, which is in the form of calories, macronutrients and micronutrients, gives your body the **fuel** to govern all the life-sustaining functions. As part of this processing, the good stuff you need is absorbed and utilized, and what it doesn't need (toxins and waste products) is then packaged up in a convenient export-shipping item called, **poop**. This is a very efficient design, in with the good and out with the bad.

This awesome design works optimally by eating what nature designed for you. In real world terms, this means eating foods designed for humans. Foods that stimulate your body to work properly.

What happens to your body when you do not feed the correct foods? Eating things that were not designed for you is how you get stuck on the hamster wheel of poor health.

This is how crash and burn happens!

A poor diet filled with non-human food items bombards your body with all sorts of by-products, chemicals, and junk that will drag your health down. These non-food items starve your body of nutrients, alter your body's proper functions, cause inflammation, and impair your ability to eliminate toxic waste effectively. Toxic waste will stay in your body longer than it should and you end up re-absorbing many harmful toxins into your bloodstream and re-circulating them in your body. This makes you and your systems **toxic**.

A toxic condition on a cumulative basis causes your entire body **stress**. All of your systems are affected. Your mental clarity, your energy levels, your weight, your hormone productions, **everything** becomes immersed in a **toxic mix**.

There is no possible way you can "lose" unhealthy weight and feel good on a permanent basis when you are in a toxic state.

Once a toxic environment starts within your body, the internal wisdom starts sending you error messages. These messages are what all of us doctors call **signs and symptoms** or **warning signs**.

Many of these "warning signs" include being overweight, high blood pressure, high cholesterol, acid-reflux, colitis, fatigue, chronic back pain, headaches, etc. These conditions are really symptoms of your body reacting to being under stress and breaking down.

I am amazed our health care industry has developed "disease" names for these warning signals. For example: acid-reflux "disease." That is like saying your car has "lack-o-gas disease" when you are low on fuel and the gaslight comes on in your car. How idiotic is that?

You don't have enough gas in the car. That is why the warning light came on. Just like your car, your body fires off a warning light when something is wrong. Acid reflux is actually a natural response to you eating something that you should not have eaten. Chronic acid reflux is telling you that you are continuing to eat things that are killing you and your system is out of balance, toxic and screaming for help. So, like the gas light in the car, your body fires a warning light to help you.

Taking a medication that suppresses your "warning light" makes as much sense as disconnecting the gaslight when you are low on gas. Yet, this is the approach we are told is effective treatment.

One hour of TV commercials full of drug ads propagate more incorrect information about human physiology than I ever thought possible. Suppress your "warning lights" long enough and you will be in a world of hurt. You can permanently fix acid-reflux "disease" as quickly as you can fix your "lack-o-gas" problem in your car. But like your car, you must put the **correct fuel** into your body in order for it to run properly. Most health conditions can be fixed by getting the appropriate **fuel**, otherwise known as proper nutrients. This has been proven time and time again in the medical literature.

It is important to remember, conditions such as obesity, chronic fatigue, anxiety, and high blood pressure could all fall under the 'Warning Light" symptoms of the body breaking down—"Warning" you that your body is living in and losing a toxic war.

Feeding your body improperly on a daily basis is like every creation of debt, it catches up with you and the interest is compounding daily. Your body does not operate well in a toxic state. It can "survive" but it cannot excel.

As it turns out, your "**diet"** is the major step in which you can take charge, correct and improve your health. There is no magic pill, no wonder juice in a bottle or no shaman smoke on earth that will return you to a state of good health and well being. Sorry, great marketing ideas, but nature is not on board with those schemes.

How do you really and truly improve your health?

Each day, you will make several choices of what to eat and put into your body. **You control** your own eating choices. This is the biggest opportunity you have every single day to enhance your health. Your body is a willing participant on your road to health. It was designed to take very good care of you. But you must be a active partner in this and help yourself by feeding your body **real food**!

When you start feeding your body with what it truly needs, you can reverse your body's breakdown and your body will love you for it. You will lose weight, feel stronger, have more energy, and the chronic symptoms of **toxic** system overload will alleviate. No more crashing and burning.

The Big Picture Ideas of how your body works:

- **Healing is a process and does take some time.**
- **Trust nature; it is on your side.**
- **Your body and your immune system know exactly how to regain and improve your health.**
- **You have the opportunity to enhance your health every single day by simply eating your way to better health.**

Now that we have covered how your body works, I must address some aspects of healing that most likely will occur. When you make the wonderful commitment to eating a more nutrient-rich diet and start applying solid nutrition into your life, your body will start working more effectively and efficiently. One of the first things your system goes through is a "Spring Cleaning." What I mean is, since you were probably not feeding yourself very well to begin with, your body is accustomed to the survival mode and not the flourishing mode. When the body is stimulated to increase healing, and that is what an infusion of high nutrients will do, all of your processing improves and out goes a lot of the toxins that have been stored in your body.

This is a good thing. However, the exiting of these toxins is not a quiet, tip-toe out when everyone is asleep kind of process. Your body, when stimulated by proper nutrients, will start to work like a hummingbird on a triple-shot latte. It will ramp up your immune system and clean house. You may experience a few symptoms that are associated with this improved performance. The good news is that these symptoms are temporary, benign, and generally occur and resolve within the first couple weeks. Common ones reported are headaches, mood swings, energy shifts, bad breath, temporary abdominal bloating and gas that can peel paint.

Some of these symptoms may have you thinking, "**I can't do this.**" But hang in there. These symptoms are common and normal. It's your body's way of correcting problems and working more efficiently. When you ask for positive changes, the universe will answer, but will also test your conviction as to how serious you are to make this wonderful transformation. Healing is a process, so have a little patience.

I cannot emphasize this enough: **Trust Nature**. Our healthcare world is polarized by diagnosis and conditions. But this is just a snapshot as to what is going on with your health at any given time. Remember that you are a living being with a wonderful innate ability to heal and be well. When given the appropriate nutrients, your body will heal and improve the quality of your life. I have never seen a patient's poor health caused by a prescription drug deficiency. Most health conditions and diseases happen slowly over time—over time without the appropriate nutrients. It does not matter what your condition is, you, as a living being, must obtain the correct nutrients to prosper and resolve health issues. And you get these nutrients from **food**.

It is bizarre when you think about most of the drug ads on TV. They all describe a drug that will alleviate the misery you are experiencing from your system not working properly. For instance, think of irregularity, otherwise known as constipation. Approximately 70% of your immune system is inside your intestinal tract, therefore your intestinal tract is important to your overall health. Constipation is a common condition as millions suffer from an inability to poop regularly. This is a real bummer, not only does it cause you discomfort, but constipation poisons you from the inside. Waste is supposed to flow through you, elminating toxins. Constipation, which is almost entirely due to eating stuff that was not designed for your system, will make you sick. How will a drug change the reoccurring problem of eating incorrect foods? It won't and it never will.

When you eat more nutrient rich foods, your elimination ability will improventhen you can "eliminate" the drugs you are using to help make you poop.

CHAPTER 2

What is Food? The misconceptions are deadly!

I started to understand the **misconceptions** many people have about "what food is" many years ago. I learned a valuable lesson as a young doctor by one of my most sincere and candid patients. I was trying to explain to this gentleman named Walt, how he needed to improve his eating habits. Walt was a tough, rugged type of man who worked in the logging business. So he got a little ticked off at me and said "Doc, I eat healthy, I eat food, what the hell are you talking about?" Then I chimed in with, "Well, if you do eat healthy and you are eating real **food**, then what's with the 30 extra pounds, reoccurring headaches, and feet that smell like you have a dead animal in your shoes?" Walt then asked me with a stern look on his face, "You can smell my feet from where you're standing?" I said, "No Walt, *everyone* could smell them from the waiting room." Then we both laughed to the point of tears and that patient visit was a great learning lesson for me as a young clinician. I then had a grasp on part of the problem. **We are confused** as to what to eat and what food really is.

"Yeah, Doc, I eat real food, so what the hell are you talking about?"

Walt got me thinking and I started to do a lot of research. This was back in 1991, long before the onslaught of genetic modified foods entered our food supply. However, even back then, non-food items had entered our lives, and as each year passed, more and more stuff was replacing actual food.

In my opinion, we have a profound misunderstanding of what food and "healthy" eating is due to the market share dominance by major food manufacturers. The bottom line is, our American nutritional guidelines and dietary information are dominated by market share and politics, **not** logic or scientific evidence. The American population is well-marketed and strategically brainwashed via the powerful commercial food industry, media, lobbyists, et al, which makes our population confused, and at times, fearful to make long-term positive changes. Just one news headline full of cow dung can set back years of scientific evidence. Yes, we have been sold out for profit and greed, only to be left in a state of poor health. This day in age, that probably shouldn't come as a complete shock to you.

However, there is a wonderful solution that has been here all along. Let me explain what **food** truthfully is and where you can easily find it. You will also discover, **real food** actually tastes great and is very easy to prepare. In many cases, you don't have to do anything to it, just eat it. How awesome is that?

I find the biggest dietary misconception is what is a **food** and what is a **product**. There is a huge difference between the two. Life and death, if you will.

As I established in Chapter 1, you need energy via nutrients for good health, and your body gets nutrients from only one source, which is food. However, we have been told that food manufacturers "make food." Ahhh, here lies the problem. **Nature makes food. Companies make products. Companies do not make food!** The food manufacturing industry makes products out of chemicals and/or **refines** nature's foods into a product, period!

Important: Our healthy fuel for life comes from food, not from products or refined foods. So where does food come from?

Food initially starts with the primary energy source for all living beings, which is the **Sun**. The Sun sends down its life-giving energy, and plants absorb this energy and convert it to oxygen and nutrients within the plant itself. We then get this transfer of energy through eating plants **directly**, or secondarily through eating animals that have first consumed plants.

Energy from the Sun

↓

To Plants

↓

Photosynthesis

↳ **{Chlorophyll rich nutrients created in the plants}**

↓

Consumed by Humans for optimal life and health = ☺

That is the simplified explanation, but that is how it works. This cannot be duplicated in a factory using chemicals, flavor enhancers, preservatives or modification of DNA.

Emotionally Charged Misconceptions; Dogma, Drama & Labels: When it comes to eating for health, you should focus on foods that give you the most nutrients without added health risks. **The best sources of nutrient-rich foods for humans are plant-based.** I am not on a political crusade for any dogma or agenda, but this is a fact-based truth. The scientific and clinical evidence is too over-whelming to ignore. Clinical evidence is showing that chronic disease is directly influenced by what we eat. Nutritional science confirms a diet rich in plant-based foods promotes good health without the added health risks that animal and processed foods contain. Diet discussions can be an emotional topic. We have been indoctrinated since birth to the myths and hype of the Standard American Diet and letting go of these misconceptions can be difficult. However, any argument perpetuating a diet consisting of foods KNOWN to cause illness and disease is truly absurd in this day and age. Many people will justify any concept to protect their eating habits. Truth, experience, empirical evidence be damned. However, you need to forget dogma, drama and labels. The argument about what dietary label you are; omnivore, blood-type, meat-eater, etc, ignores human physiology. Your body is governed by physiological processes which requires nutrients and it does not care about dogma, drama & labels.

You must not forget that you are a living being; therefore, eating plant-based foods, which are unprocessed and naturally balanced from nature, is ideal for your system. Vegetables, fruits, beans, nuts, seeds, and grains contain the comprehensive nutrients needed for good health. They also contain anti-oxidants and phytonutrients designed to strengthen your immune system and help prevent diseases. A diet of nutrient-rich plant-based sources is the **food** for human health. (Chapter 5 covers nutritional needs.)

It is important to understand your "diet" is the cornerstone of your health. No two ways about it. Now, don't get confused with the "diet" industry word, which is something you may "go on" for a specific goal, like to lose weight because you bought a smaller size pair of pants to motivate you. I am talking about what you NEED to eat to be healthy. Remember the word **diet** or "a way of life" means your dietary requirements you must obtain through eating foods to keep your body healthy and happy. For you to enjoy success in all aspects of your health, you must choose **food** more often than you choose products.

> Remember this little mantra:
>
> **"Food is made by nature. Products are made by companies."**

The key to remember when you are contemplating whether it is a food or a product is what is done to it before it gets into your hands. For example, most every plant-based food such as kale, broccoli, spinach, garlic, apples, or oranges can be eaten **raw** in their natural state without cooking or processing. This applies to nearly all plant-based food items on earth. All of the vital nutrients; anitoxidants, vitamins, minerals and phytonutrients are already in the food and you don't need to add anything. Beans and grains such as brown rice require simple cooking in boiling water to make them ready to consume. So, if it took a host of caustic chemicals to get it into a little box so it can sit on a shelf for a year or you have to cook it at high heat for an hour to avoid sickness or death due to bacteria or parasites then it is a **product**, **not food**.

If you still have a question as to what is a food, think of where nature would have safely and securely placed our nutrients for us to survive and flourish throughout time. Yes, once again, it's plants. Humans have been walking the earth long before the art of cooking, processing, freezing, or microwaving was invented.

5 Key Points to Remember About Food:

1. **Food is made by nature not by companies.**
2. **You were made by nature not by companies.**
3. **Food is a requirement your body needs each day.**
4. **Food is what your body is designed to eat.**
5. **Trust nature's design:**

   Nature created comprehensive nutritional gifts in the form of healing plant foods called vegetables, fruits, nuts, seeds and grains. They are nutrient-rich, unprocessed and designed for your system.

Definitions:

Raw: I use the term raw to define plant-based food in its most natural state, meaning uncooked, unprocessed, virtually untouched before it comes to you. Other terms used in the raw food industry are "living foods" or "live foods."

Diet: Unless specifically speaking of a "diet" regimen, I refer to diet as to the food choices you make to sustain and enhance your life and health. From the definition of the word diet, diaita, which means "a way of life."

Fortified: Due to the high-refinement and chemical processing used in the conventional food manufacturing industry over the past several decades, "fortified"—techniques of adding vitamins and minerals into the processed product—has been used to replace the nutrients that were lost in processing. This is not ideal for human consumption or health. However, you will see many good, responsible natural food companies fortify their products like nut milks and cereals for added health benefits. So fortified does not always mean that the item has been overly-processed. As you become more familiar with the good, ethical natural food companies, you will see, understand, and taste the difference.

Summary of Food or Products:

Our lifestyles have become so fast-paced that we are now a society of convenience. If it is not quick and easy, then it is not happening. But nuking a box of pre-assembled synthetic non-food items to save time does not promote good health. Nor will it address why your health is falling apart. And guess what? When your health is in the crapper, there is no 2-minute "high" setting button to push to restore it either. I find many people have a misconception of how quick and easy preparing real food actually is. It is easy to accomplish and you will **feel** the wonderful difference. My design doesn't prevent you from having some of your old favorite items, even if they are from a box. My design will show you the difference between real food and products, and how you can close the gap, enjoy great food, restore your health, and still be you.

CHAPTER 3

Diet: Food Is Not Your Enemy!

In the quest for better health, most everyone has tried a “diet” or two. Some of you have spent a lifetime off and on diets. As a doctor, what really ticks me off is how the diet industry preys upon people’s hopes to lose weight.

The diet industry and most weight loss gurus tell you their “diet” will help you lose weight quickly. As an example, something like “lose 30 pounds in 2 weeks.” Now in all fairness, what they did say is “lose weight.” That is the hook that gets anyone who wants to lose weight suckered in. But, you don’t just want to lose weight. You want to burn fat and you want to feel better. You want more energy and you want to look great in those new clothes.

The fundamental problem with “diets” is they are weight loss-driven, not health-driven. You "go on" a diet, experience a little weight loss, then your body rebounds from the shock of the unsound “diet” design and your weight returns, often times with additional pounds.

So you blame yourself for not having the willpower to stick with it. However, you were not the problem. The “diet” was the problem. But now your self-esteem is dinged and you are more frustrated than ever.

Think of dieting like this: If I told you to drive from San Francisco to Los Angeles (about 400 miles) on a half a tank of gas, you would run out of gas halfway there. You also would not be mad at yourself. You would be cussing my name and buying a ticket back home to strangle me. Justifiably so, as I told you to do something that was impossible. It is the same with dieting. Most “diets” are physiologically unsound. If you need proof, I am sure you have tried many with fleeting results, only to be left where you were initially or in worse shape before you started.

The only thing that lost weight was your wallet from the money you spent on a bad diet design.

When a patient tells me they want to lose weight, I know what they are saying. They want to lose fat, not just weight. Your body is very capable of burning the fat and slimming down to your biological structure with ease; it just needs the correct program.

A note on biological structure:

If you are of a larger build, don't try to get down to a size 0. We humans are built in all shapes and sizes. But even if you were born a "bigger" person, your natural, lean, low body fat, high energetic shape will be very appealing to you, I promise, even if you never make it down to be a size 0.

I am 6'2" and I wear a 42 long jacket. Trying to wear a 38 jacket may make me look more "buffed" but I will also look like I am wearing children's clothes. Not the look I need.

To get where you want to be with your weight, **you must** first stabilize your entire system. This is the **only** way to burn **fat** and lose the excess weight. As I pointed out in Chapter 1, if your body is toxic, your system is impaired. **You CANNOT ask your body to burn fat** while your body is living in a toxic state. This is why "diets" don't work. They never address the toxic status of your health and many "diets" can create more toxicity for you.

The same is similar for other conditions such as thyroid conditions. Many people are lead to believe a hormonal disturbance, particularly their thyroid, is the main reason they are overweight. Yes, hormonal problems, including thyroid, can cause the body to have weight problems. However, being put on life long medication does not fix their weight issues. Many patients I have treated with thyroid conditions respond well to my diet protocols and do not have to continue with the life long medications. With the implementation of eating real food more often, they are no longer on the "diet" roller coaster.

Their body starts to work more efficiently and balance is restored. These patients enjoy permanent weight loss, more energy and feel better overall. You must improve your body's processing ability. That is the key to health. The "diet" industry is a multi-billion dollar a year industry and they sell weight loss. They actually promise and for the short-term deliver weight loss. But they are smart enough **not** to claim fat-loss or health benefits. By understanding the diet industry is just that, an industry and not a health solution, you will have success in reaching your goal of getting healthier.

As living beings, nature did not design us to be overweight, lethargic beings. We all have the biological blueprint to be lean, healthy people. We do come in all shapes and sizes, that is true, but to be overweight, sluggish and chronically feeling fatigued is not our genetic makeup. That is a direct result of our gluttony of poor dietary habits and misconceptions of how to eat properly.

This also holds true for those of you who reduce your calories to be thin. When you significantly restrict your calories, your body is in a constant state of nutrient bankruptcy and you are paying the bill with your health, literally. You may be thin and you may be at the "weight" you desire, but I am willing to bet you have the same toxic issues of headaches, low energy, and mood swings as you did before, and it is an everyday fight to stay thin. Good health is not a state of being overweight or starving to be thin. Good health is achieved by eating nutrient-rich foods. Also, having a month supply of "food" shipped to you in a box is definitely a system, but not a nutrient-based system. It is just another absurd idea intent on getting you to buy something with the hope of losing weight. Locking you in a closet for the weekend would make you lose weight, too, but I don't advise that either.

A note on Diet "Flushes" of all kinds:

There are many "detox" fat flushes/diets out there. Please be careful. Most of the flushes marketed are diuretic-based and you end up losing large amounts of water weight, minerals and electrolytes. Flush concoctions, laxatives and even appetite suppressive products can never be substituted for your nutritional needs. To truly "detox" your system, simply start the process of eating better. Your body knows how to take care of you. You make simple and effective changes to clean up your diet and your health improves, you lose weight and have more energy. You cannot go wrong by eating foods from nature, so if it smells like something else, it probably is. Don't step in it, and for goodness sake, **don't eat it**!

Key Points to Remember about Dieting:

1. **Most "diets" promise weight-loss, not fat-loss or improved health.**
2. **Most "diets" cause roller coaster effects in your weight, your health and your sanity.**
3. **Calorie restriction, starving yourself, or exerting more guilt onto yourself is not the path to becoming healthier.**
4. **In the past, when the unsound "diet design" broke down and the short-term results were gone, you took the blame as not having the desire, will power or effort to succeed.**
5. **Do not blame yourself for being preyed upon and following a bad design. You are human, it happens and a unsound diet design is not your fault.**
6. **Diet actually means a way of life. Therefore, eating the way your body was designed will create the way of life you want. Healthy, leaner, more energy with better mental clarity.**

CHAPTER 4

Inflammation: Killing You From the Inside Out

Inflammation is a important subject because it can have a negative effect on your health. That is why this entire chapter is dedicated to helping you understand inflammation.

In the medical community, we now have a better understanding of how chronic inflammation plays a significant role in poor health. It is becoming increasingly clear that a host of illnesses, such as heart disease, many cancers, autoimmune syndromes, even Alzheimer's are influenced in large part by chronic inflammation. Chronic inflammation is a process in which the immune system becomes out of balance and continually tries to repair the body and repel pathogens. Chronic inflammation will damage your healthy tissues as well. Stress, lack of exercise, genetic predisposition and other poor lifestyle choices can all promote inflammation, but a poor diet is the main culprit. Many people perpetuate their chronic inflammation every single day by simply eating and drinking stuff that stimulates the inflammatory process.

There are many "anti-inflammatory" diet books published with all sorts of suggestions to reduce inflammation, but I find most people do not understand the **source** of what is causing their inflammation.

Inflammation is a very important process. It is actually a tool your immune system uses to fight off infections and repair injuries. Inflammation is needed and necessary. It is what clots your blood when you have a cut and arrives like a medic to an area of infection when called to do so.

Inflammation can be broken into two main terms:

1. Acute Inflammation
2. Chronic Inflammation

A simplified definition for **Acute inflammation** is: "Acute inflammation is a *short-term* process which is characterized by the classic signs of inflammation—swelling, redness, pain, heat, and loss of function." Acute inflammation is triggered by harmful stimuli or an injury, like when you twist your ankle.

Chronic inflammation can be summed up as: "Chronic inflammation is a **pathological condition**, characterized by concurrent active inflammation, tissue destruction, and attempts at repair."

Chronic inflammation is actually destructive to your entire system. Chronic inflammation is **prolonged inflammation** and is the acute inflammatory response **over and over** on a recurring basis. All of your tissues are affected; your heart, liver, blood vessels, even your psyche must deal with chronic inflammation. Chronic inflammation is a killer.

This is the **concept** part many people do not fully understand. Since the inflammation is occurring on a repeated, continual basis, it is important to understand that you have an active role in this process. Many people are creating the inflammatory response within their body everyday with poor eating choices, but they do not realize where it is coming from.

There are many things on this planet that can be a harmful stimuli to your body. If you go back to Chapter 1, remember acid-reflux. That is a full blown inflammatory response to you eating something harmful to your system and your body is fighting to deal with it.

Your body will react to **anything and everything** it sees as a harmful threat. That is its job. Getting hit by a baseball traveling at high speed will create inflammation. That is fairly easy to understand. However, eating toxic items, such as artificial **sweeteners, food dyes, preservatives, trans-fats and even animal flesh and animal body fluids like cow's milk can cause inflammation**.

By eating inflammatory-stimulating items on a **daily basis**, your body will respond **appropriately** by launching the inflammation process. Eating items that stimulate inflammation daily, your body will get overwhelmed with chronic inflammation and good health will be harder to achieve. This will also give you an overall uneasy feeling; a feeling that something is just not right. Chronic pain, headaches, fatigue, bloating and swelling are common complaints of inflammation.

> Eating items not designed for you by nature will stimulate an immune response (inflammation) to protect your systems.
>
> If you are eating items that are causing inflammation, your body must go into the defense mode and neutralize the harmful stimuli you consumed. In the defense mode, your body is busy fighting, not flourishing.

The following list of items cause inflammation and create toxicity in the body. These items are commonly consumed daily by many people who don't give it much thought, however, these items are not good for you. Once in a while maybe OK; however, if you are eating a lot of this stuff each week, I am sure they are creating problems for you.

Items that can elicit the toxic/inflammatory response:

- **Refined/Processed Sugars and Flour Products:** Examples are white rice, white pastas, refined sweets, and pastries. These processed food products are stripped of nutrients and saturated with chemicals due to processing. Most every highly processed boxed, microwavable, instant "food" products contain these toxic items.

- **Animal Flesh and Fluids: Meats & Dairy:** Contrary to market generated ideas, there is **no human dietary requirement for the flesh or body fluids from animals**. These substances were designed for true carnivores. Examples of the **flesh** are red meat, chicken, pork, fish, etc. **The fluids:** animal breast milk, cheese, and milk products of any and all sorts. Yes, they can and do promote inflammation in humans.
- **Preservatives:** Chemicals used to keep a product around a long time on the shelf. Great for companies, not for your health.
- **Artificial Flavorings:** Chemicals designed to mimic real food flavors. Nature holds the patent for wonderful real food flavors and nutrients. Stay with the patent holder and you cannot go wrong.
- **Conventionally Grown Produce:** Fruits and vegetables that have been grown with synthetic toxic compounds. Anything that can kill a cockroach, you do not want to eat if possible.
- **Genetically Modified Organism (GMO's):** Food items manipulated by companies for various reasons, profit being #1. DNA manipulation is generally *not* a good idea, so to eat something that has been altered in a lab is not a good idea either.
- **Medications/Drugs:** Some prescription and over the counter medications can promote inflammation within the body due to their chemical structure. If you are following the advice of your doctor by using meds, all the more reason to eat a healthier diet rich with foods designed for your body's systems. You may find you will no longer need the drugs when eating better.
- **Alcohol:** Consistent over use of alcohol is a stimulus of inflammation. Red wine appears to have antioxidant properties but not in excessive amounts.

Keep the Real World Big Picture:

Life is cumulative and so is your diet. I understand there are many "junk" items people don't want to give up. It's my goal to help you understand how to eat better without eliminating all the junkie items you love.

There are many synthetic items added into food products that are **highly toxic**, yet we overlook them or do not know much about them. I advise you to read the list of **avoid** items in Appendix C: Product Ingredients to Avoid at the back of the book, then read labels when shopping and try to avoid these toxins. If you clean up your food supply by eliminating unnecessary poisons, your body will be happier. While the list above might have knocked many of the items you currently enjoy, my **16/21 Diet Solution** will still allow you plenty of room to enjoy your life. For many of you, it will show you a door to a wonderful world of great-tasting real food you may never knew existed. If you follow my recommendations, you will have good results. So don't worry, just stay on the path.

Misinformation is everywhere; therefore my goal is to point out items that really hamper your path to better health. Chronic inflammation can be reduced and eliminated with a solid healthy diet. **16/21** delivers this for you. Those of you who think you are "fat"; it is quite possible that you are not all that "fat" but systemically bloated from toxic items. This overweight state is from chronic inflammation, which causes excessive fluid retention and weight gain. Cleaner eating resolves the inflammation so the body can then move on to burning fat. Once again, another win-win scenario.

I see a similar problem with chronic pain patients. Many patients ask me what physical activity they should stop doing to reduce their pain. However, a large part of the problem is coming from eating items each and every day that inflame their system and causes pain with *all* types of movements, not one in particular. Cleaning up your diet, will clean up your system and decrease your pain!

Key Points to Remember about Inflammation:

- You can inadvertently create inflammation on a daily basis by eating items that are not designed for your body.
- Daily and continual consumption of inflammatory promoting items cause an immune system reaction, creating chronic inflammation. Chronic inflammation accelerates poor health and pre-maturely ages you inside and out.
- Chronic inflammation can keep you feeling bloated, fatigued, and can give you an overall "heavy" tired feeling.
- It is possible that you have been looking at yourself as fat when you may be more toxic and bloated, the signs of inflammation. I have treated many overweight patients that were not all that high in body fat when measured. However, they were heavy and literally carrying around a lot of extra weight and size due to their chronic swollen tissues. Looking and feeling "fat" may be due to chronic inflammation more then just being fat.
- Your body can handle and eliminate inflammation and the symptoms of toxic living with the correct foods.
- 16/21 is structured to help you return to a leaner, less toxic, less inflamed state of living.

CHAPTER 5

Your Real Nutritional Needs: Don't Make It So Dang Hard

Another confusing concept for people is their nutritional needs. I understand why it is so confusing, as once again, market share, the Internet, TV commercials and that crazy uncle are infused with not so accurate information.

This chapter will outline what you "need" on a nutritional basis, how much and where to get it. Once again, I want you to keep the Big Picture Idea.

7 Things You Need for Optimum Health:

1. **Carbohydrates**
2. **Adequate Protein**
3. **Fats**
4. **Vitamins/Minerals**
5. **Fiber**
6. **Phytonutrients**
7. **Fresh Water**

Caloric Requirements: Most adults need to consume between 1,800 and 2,800 calories a day. Once you eat to heal and strengthen your body as outlined in the **16/21 Diet Solution**, your weight should not fluctuate greatly. You do not need to drive yourself nuts trying to count calories. You will find nutrient rich foods are not high in calories anyway.

So, there is no need to stress about caloric intake. Try to include carbohydrates, fat, and protein at each meal. Don't make it rocket science; understand the concepts in this book as to what your body needs. Eat those foods most of the time, relax and enjoy.

For those of you who love ratios, your diet is at a good balance when you eat: 60-70% complex carbs, 15-20% protein, 15-20% fats. Remember, if you are eating real foods (see Chapter 2: What is Food?), you are doing just fine.

Put it into perspective with this thought: "Nutrients are what my body needs for health and vitality."

1. Carbohydrates:

Your body burns carbohydrates as its primary fuel. You need carbs for energy, metabolic activities, neurological functions, and repair. Your body looks to burn carbohydrates in the form of glucose as the first choice for fuel. Therefore, your diet must include sufficient carbs. If you do not eat a sufficient supply of carbs in your diet, your body will steal glucose from your muscles for fuel. (Living muscle tissue is mostly blood, glucose, and water.) This accounts for the large amount of weight loss in low carb diets. However, this is detrimental for your health. As I tell my kids, "Stealing never pays off." So stealing fuel from within your body does not promote health.

Carbohydrates are talked about in two forms:

- Complex Carbs (example: whole grains)
- Simple Sugars (example: fruits)

Complex carbs burn slower over time and give the body a nice, sustained energy source without the spikes. Simple sugars are just that, simple. Fruits contain simple sugars and burn fairly quickly, but are still a good source of energy, as they also are packed full of nutrients.

Your body is designed to eat a mixture of complex and simple carbs. These are the natural sugars that nature designed for you.

The Carbohydrate Confusion: Let's Clarify

Remember, **nature** built 2 Types of Carbohydrates:

1). Complex, like whole grains.

2). Simple, like fruit.

Refined, processed foods such as white breads, white rice, white pastas, and sugars are not foods. They are not complex or simple sugars. They are processed man-made products and they are toxic.

Do not think of "refined" foods as food. Think of them as "junk" as they do not contain any health-enhancing properties.

The refining process strips most every nutrient and fiber from the food. The package label will tell you this. If it states, "*enriched* flour" on the ingredient list, that tells you immediately that you are *not* eating food. You are eating a heavily refined product being passed passed off as food. Plus, refining is done with caustic chemicals and you ingest these toxins with your meal. (Think chronic inflammation—bad news!) Therefore you can forget the entire carb argument and the nutritional value stated on the package. **Refined** products contribute to **inflammation**, **obesity** and many other diseases. They are not carbs, they are junk. Period!

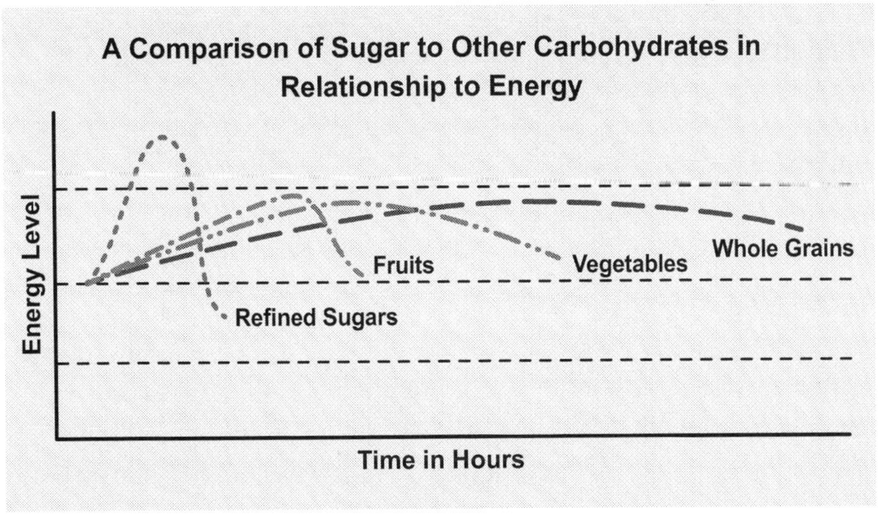

Refined sugars will spike and crash your energy level, while fruit, vegetable and whole grain sugars burn more evenly throughout the day.

Nature's carbs, in the form of **whole foods**, burn better in your system, provide sustained energy, and do not make you fat. **Refined products** have been linked to many diseases such as: Cancers of the stomach, intestinal tract, breast, thyroid and colorectal regions, as well as diabetes, gallbladder problems and heart disease. Refined sugars include sucrose (table sugar), lactose (milk sugar), brown sugar, high-fructose corn syrup, corn sweetener, and concentrated fruit juices. No nutritional value, but highly toxic to you, especially to kids.

Also, be careful of products labeled "whole grain." It may have a little whole grain flour, but still may contain toxic processed sugars, GMO's and/or chemical stabilizers. Once again, buyer beware of tricky marketing.

The Skinny on Low-Carb Dieting:

There are numerous clinical studies showing patients who eat a diet low in carbs and high in protein, particularly animal proteins, have a poorer state of health than those who eat fresh fruits, vegetables and whole grains. By eating a low-carb diet, you are restricting your body from high nutrient-based foods and energy sources you need for health. Therefore, your initial loss of weight was not permanent and due to the high amount of animal proteins and fat, your risk of dying of the number one killer in the U.S., heart disease, went up dramatically.

2. Protein:

Protein is needed for growth, repair and immunity. However, the building blocks of protein are Amino Acids. You require amino acids to make your body's protein. The majority of amino acids are made within your body. However, there are 9 "essential" amino acids. They are called essential, as your body cannot make them; therefore these 9 essential amino acids must come from the foods you eat. Amino acids are easy to get as they are found in all living cells both plant and animal.

<u>Too Much Protein is Not Good for You</u>: (The Protein Myth)

Our food supply is dominated by protein producing companies. So guess what? These companies are going to work hard to convince you that a lot of protein is needed and anything going wrong with you is because you are lacking their protein laced products. Within the Standard American Diet (SAD), the average person consumes double the daily requirement for protein. To compound this problem, the majority of protein consumed is derived from animal sources. Animal sources are high in **unhealthy fat and cholesterol**. It is well documented, the over consumption of proteins and specifically animal protein, shows a direct link to health conditions such as:

- **Cardiovascular Disease (heart disease)**
- **Impaired kidney function**
- **Osteoporosis**
- **Cancers of the brain, breast, colon, intestines, leukemia, lymphoma, ovaries, pancreas, prostate and stomach.**

For anyone who is athletic, especially growing teenagers who want bigger muscles, eating excessive amounts of protein does not make your muscles bigger. But it will set you up for future health problems. This is a prime example of **more is not better**! In fact, many teenage student athletes are using protein powders that are extremely high in protein load for their bodies. Too much protein hurts the body's performance and overall health.

Look at it this way: If you filled a 10-gallon gas can with 15 gallons of gas, 5 gallons would spill out and make a dangerous mess. This holds true for protein consumption too. You do need protein but not in excess. Excessive protein is **toxic** to your entire system. Protein deficiency is extremely rare in developed countries however cancers and other degenerative diseases are the leading cause of death. Correlation???.......Absolutely!!

I find it irresponsible for doctors and nutritional "experts" to perpetuate the out dated and mythical idea that high protein intake is beneficial. The clinical evidence and scientific scrutiny states the contrary and the consequences are dangerous.

Myth: You need animal proteins because they are "complete" proteins. Plant proteins lack essential amino acids and are not complete.

Fact: Plant-based foods provide an abundant source of essential amino acids and provide complete proteins.

If you have been told that you must eat an animal's flesh or fluids for protein, ask yourself, where did the large muscular animal you think you "must" eat get its protein?
That's Right, from plants! The animals you are eating are *vegetarian*!

Protein Intake:

An estimator used for daily protein intake is **0.36 grams per 1 pound** of body weight. For example, if you weigh 155 lbs. X .36 = 56 grams per day. **But if you are overweight to begin with, do not use this estimator** for your current body weight because this will calculate a higher protein intake number than you really need and you will perpetuate your health problems.

A healthy daily protein intake guideline: (I prefer this chart)

Daily Protein Intake Guidelines:

Males (14 yrs +)	50-75 grams
Female (14 yrs +)	45-60 grams
Pregnant Female (Breast-feeding Mommies too)	70-85 grams
Children:	
1-3 yrs	15-20 grams
4-8 yrs	22-25 grams
9-13 yrs	35-45 grams

Pregnant and breast-feeding women do need a higher amount of protein. But they also need a higher amount of nutrients, not just protein. Eating more unrefined nutrient rich foods is the key. You do not have to double the recommended daily amount of protein.

The never-ending question: "If you want me to reduce meat in my diet, where will I get my protein?" Remember, it is amino acids you need from your diet. Your body extracts amino acids from the protein in the food you eat to build your own protein. Eating meat for the protein also gives you a large quantity of fat and cholesterol with each bite. Green vegetables and beans are especially full of protein. The largest animals in the world (elephants, rhinos and horses) are complete vegetarians. Therefore, it is evident that plant-based foods are packed with all the amino acids you need, too. The true carnivore (tiger) gets nutrients by eating vegetarian animals. The tiger has the **ability** to eat raw, unprocessed meat, ligaments, blood, bone and brain tissue of its prey since animal parts are the natural food source of carnivores. We don't eat meat or animal tissue anything like a real carnivore. We eat cadaver meat; body parts of animals killed weeks or months prior to consumption, after it is treated, preserved or enhanced for flavor. This is not "all natural," nor does it even make sense. Wild animals will not eat meat that has been lying around for many days.

Plant-Based Protein Foods:

- Almond Butter, 2 T — 5 grams
- Broccoli, 1 cup — 5 grams
- Cashews, 1/4 cup — 5 grams
- Kale, 1 cup — 3 grams
- Seitan, 4 oz — 15 grams
- Soy Milk 8 oz — 6 grams
- Tahini, 1 T — 3 grams
- Tofu 6 oz — 20 grams
- Black Beans, 1 cup — 15 grams
- Brown Rice, 1 cup — 5 grams
- Garbanzos 1 cup — 15 grams
- Lentils, 1 cup — 18 grams
- Quinoa, 1 cup — 10 grams
- Spinach, 1 cup — 6 grams
- Tempeh, 3 oz — 22 grams
- Whole Grain Bread, 1 slice — 4 grams

Yes, I have included recipes made with all of these quality protein foods, don't worry. ☺

Plant-based proteins contain additional health goodies:

Plants contain fiber, anti-oxidants and phytonutrients, providing added protective benefits to your health. Doctors everywhere are preaching the health benefits and disease prevention properties of fiber, anti-oxidants and phytonutrients, as research is showing they are essential to health and immune system function. However, these health gifts are **only found** in nutrient-rich plant-based foods, such as vegetables, beans, fruits, nuts and seeds. Devouring dead carcass (meats) with the thought of "getting your protein" increases your risk of the top killers of our population with no true added health benefit.

3. Fats:

There is a lot of confusion with respect to fats and health. First off, fats are essential for the body. The body uses fats in many metabolic functions. Dietary fats are important for the transport of the fat-soluble vitamins A, D, E and K, and aid in the absorption of other vitamins, minerals and phytonutrients. Fats also play a crucial role in stabilizing blood sugar levels, the making of hormones, and contributing to a healthy immune system. There are good and bad fats. However, like carbs, there is confusion. Good fats do not make you fat! If you are eating a healthy real food diet, you do not have to be overly concerned with eating nature's fats that are found within real foods.

Bad Fats: As I have said before, animal tissue is not ideal for human consumption. It is structured for large carnivores like a tiger or great white shark. Have you ever wondered why you feel like hell after you eat a large amount of animal flesh? You were not designed for it. Animal flesh is full of fat and cholesterol, which requires a physiological design that humans do not have. There is a **huge** physiological difference between humans and carnivores. Carnivores eat large amounts of meat at one time and then don't eat for several weeks. Try that yourself and you will quickly see that you are built just like all the other plant-based consuming animals. You need to eat nearly every day and your system performs better on plant-based foods. Also, look at the marketing term "lean meats." What? If something is 28% protein and 0% carbs, that makes it 72% Fat. Sorry folks, that is not lean.

It's definitely full of bull, but that is not lean. Another brilliant marketing term designed to mislead the hungry consumer. (Remember market share dominance by the protein sellers.) Dairy milk can fall into the tricky marketing scheme, too. 2% milk is 35% fat and whole milk is 49% fat. Not a big difference, especially since milk does not do the body good. I'll cover this later. Animal tissue is also high in the *inflammatory* substance, arachidonic acid (AA). If you have chronic pain or frequent upper respiratory infections, meat and dairy is something you want to strictly limit or even omit.

Another dangerous fat that is called "fats" by the food industry, but should not be classified as a fat are **trans-fats.** Trans-fats are **chemically changed fats**. What was once natural oil, trans-fats have been radically changed via chemistry and become commercial cooking oils, as well as a major ingredient in processed foods. Trans-fats are toxic to your body and have no nutritional value. Fast-food products contain a lot of these toxic "fats," as they are cheap and have a long shelf life. Trans-fats are nasty, highly-toxic substances you should avoid like the plague. Trans-fats are also known as hydrogenated or partially hydrogenated oils. Read labels carefully.

Good Fats: The fats you need! Good fats are found in plant-based sources and will provide you the fat requirements you need without increasing your risk of poor health. Unrefined (raw) plant fats are best for health and cooking. Cold pressed plant oils are actually helpful by providing you with the essential fats you need for good health.

<u>Natural oils are fat</u>: (but that is not a bad thing)

Oils are fat by definition; but don't shy away from using them appropriately for health and for taste. You will also find that by using natural oils, you will not need to use as much as conventional oils for cooking or taste. A little bit goes a long way.

Raw (unrefined) cold-pressed plant oils are wonderful multifunctional nutrient-based helpers that also add great flavor to your meals. Oils are used in many recipes, both cooked and uncooked. Natural oils are the way to go when it comes to meal preparation. To clarify, as part of a healthy diet, it is important to eliminate or dramatically reduce any animal-based fats/oils. **Any hydrogenated oils (trans-fat oils) must be completely eliminated.** Trans-fats are not food, they are products—heavily refined, contaminated products that cause poor health. They are very toxic, damaging to your heart, internal organs and blood vessels, and stimulate inflammation within the body. I am sure you have noticed how trans fats are now being exposed and making the list of foods to avoid. Health conscious clinicians have been condemning trans-fats for twenty-plus years.

Marketing Tactic: Danger, Danger, Danger!

I have read some food product packages stating 0 grams of trans fat. That statement can be dangerous and misleading.

Realize that 999 milligrams is 1 milligram short of a gram. So for a company to say 0 grams may not mean there is no trans fat in their product. It may contain 750 milligrams, which technically is 0 grams. Be careful reading packages and advertisements. Make sure it says "No Trans Fats!"

Essential Fatty Acids:

Essential fatty acids (EFA's) play an important role in good health. Essential fatty acid talk is everywhere and the EFA market is as big as ever. I also find many people are confused as to how much and what kind of EFA's you need.

The Big Picture on Essential Fatty Acids:

Fatty acids are necessary for good health. They are especially important to your brain, nervous and immune system. Similar to the essential amino acids of protein, there are two main essential fatty acids that cannot be made by the body and must be consumed in the diet. These two play an important role in the synthesis of inflammatory & anti-inflammatory properties within the body. We require an important balance of EFA's to help maintain good health.

The two main EFA's are called omega-3 and omega-6 fatty acids. Omega-3 and omega-6 fatty acids are important for normal bodily functions. Deficiencies are responsible for a host of symptoms and disorders, including abnormalities of the liver and kidneys, changes in the blood, reduced growth rates, decreased immune function, depression, skin changes, including dryness and inflammation.

It is important these two EFA's are consumed within the diet and in a balanced setting. Omega-6 and omega-3 EFA's share a conversion enzyme in the body, therefore excessive intake of omega-6's can be problematic. The standard American diet (SAD) has become too high in omega-6 and too low in omega-3 largely due to processed foods, processed oils and animal products. It is estimated the (SAD) is 14-25 times higher in omega-6 than omega-3. Clinically, this is a problem as omega-6's promote inflammation while omega-3's help to reduce it. Remember, chronic inflammation plays a role in the disease process.

Omega-6 Fatty Acids:

Omega-6's are found in leafy vegetables, seeds, nuts, grains, and vegetable oils (ie: sesame, safflower, soybean and sunflower). Most diets provide adequate amounts of omega-6 fatty acids, so deficiency is not a concern and supplementation is usually not needed. Cutting processed food products, processed oils and animal based products out of the diet will substantially help improve the omega-3 to omega-6 ratio.

Omega-3 Fatty Acids:

Omega-3 fatty acids are also found in many vegetables, beans, nuts, seeds, and fruits. Avocados, flaxseeds, flaxseed oil, hemp oil and walnuts are high in omega-3's. Studies show increasing dietary intake of omega 3's helps to reduce chronic inflammation and the risk of heart disease, stroke and high blood pressure. Fish oils are a popular source of omega-3's due to a large marketing campaign. However, in my opinion, fish oils, like all animal products, have their hazards too.

Fish & Fish Oils May Not Be the Best:

Fish oils have been praised as good sources of omega-3 fatty acids for cardiovascular disease, joint pain and better brain function. Other studies show the contrary. In my opinion, the high amounts of fat and cholesterol make fish oils a poor choice. Additionally, fish is one of the most polluted food items consumed. The toxicity of fish is a legitimate concern and well documented, as fish are high in mercury and other environmental toxins. Government warning signs are posted where fish is sold due to these dangerous toxins. Yet fish is still marketed as a health food. You do not want to add neurotoxins to your system, or especially to growing children. Fish oils can be highly unstable and tend to decompose after processing and can unleash dangerous free radicals when consumed. The fish oil is touted due to its DHA and EPA content (part of the omega-3's nutrient family). But fish are not the original source of DHA/EPA. The original source is actually microalgae the fish eats, converts and stores inside its tissues, where it is extracted from the fish and bottled for the consumer. Research has shown the more stable omega-3's are found in vegetables, fruits, and beans. As for direct DHA/EPA sources, omega-3 supplements are an additional option. If you currently take fish oils and think they are adding benefits to your health, then you may want to stay with what you are comfortable with. However, there are some good supplements that are fish-free. The **fish-free** supplements provide the DHA/EPA components of omega-3's. *Neuromins, Spectrum's DHA,* and *Udo's Choice* unrefined algae DHA vegetarian caps are reputable supplements.

Within my 16/21 Diet Solution, there is no need to worry about getting enough omega-3's compared to omega-6's. By providing a consistent intake of fresh fruits, vegetables, nuts, seeds, grains and legumes you will enjoy the adequate intake of the essential fatty acids you need without giving it much thought.

4. Vitamins & Minerals:

Vitamins and Minerals are micronutrients your body needs. They do not contain calories nor are they a direct energy source, however they assist in metabolizing nutrients in food and are invaluable in keeping your body running smoothly.

Deficiencies can lead to poor health. The following is *not* a complete list of all required vitamins/minerals but a solid list you should be aware of. Also, the suggested foods under each vitamin/mineral are examples of foods that contain the nutrients, but not the entire list of foods that supply the specific vitamin or mineral.

Vitamins:

A: Known as the vision vitamin, Vitamin A has big anti-oxidant properties, essential for growth, repair, blood production and great for skin health (your largest organ) **Foods: Dark greens, carrots, mangos, butternut squash.**

B's: The B family is made up of: B1, B2, B6, B12, Niacin, Folic acid, Biotin, and Pantothenic acid. Important for blood production, energy conversion, nerve function, digestion, growth, repair and immunity. **Foods: Whole grains, leafy green vegetables, beans and peas, fortified cereals, meat substitute items and nut-milks. Eat kale and spinach several times per week.**

C: A powerful anti-oxidant; plays a primary role in the formation of collagen, which is important for the growth and repair of body tissue cells, gums, blood vessels, bones and teeth. Also protects against the harmful effects of pollution, protects against infection, and enhances the immune system. **Foods: Oranges, strawberries, tomatoes, broccoli, red peppers.**

D: Important in maintaining normal calcium metabolism and immune system function. Vitamin D is not found in many foods. Your body can make vitamin D from sunlight exposure; however, I do not recommend relying on sunlight alone. **The good news is most quality, pre-made food items you buy today are fortified with vitamin D. Shiitake mushrooms are also a good source.**

E: Called a "super" anti-oxidant, vitamin E protects cells against damage caused by "free-radicals" (toxins). Research has shown vitamin E to be extremely important in the prevention of cancer and cardiovascular disease. **Foods: Olive oil (raw), almonds, hazelnuts, carrots, avocados.**

K: Essential for blood clotting and immune function. **Foods: Kale, spinach, leaf lettuce, Swiss chard, broccoli, greens once again!**

Minerals:

Calcium: Calcium is an important mineral for bone growth and systemic functions. It is easy to get and is everywhere in food. Simply look where a cow gets her calcium. Yes, vegetation! The dairy industry wants you to think they are the only supplier of calcium on earth. Now do you think our Creator would have done that? How long has the dairy industry been in existence? And how long ago were humans and plants created? Yeah, do the math. Nature stocked calcium everywhere and many veggies have more bio-available calcium than milk. Organic pre-made food products in the stores are also fortified with calcium as well. **Good calcium sources are: collard greens, broccoli, kale, turnips, tofu set with calcium, pinto beans, white beans, and fortified soy/nut milk all contain high quantities of calcium. (Dark greens actually deliver the added benefit of supplying vitamins and minerals that contribute to bone health, such as vitamins C and K, folate, magnesium, potassium, and boron.)**

"Calcium killers" can negatively affect your calcium levels. Poor dietary choices, such as high sodium consumption, too much protein (especially animal sources), caffeine, and soft drinks with phosphoric acid can cause increased calcium loss. Diet sodas are very popular with women and teenage girls, but they are problematic to the calcium balance for females.

Magnesium: Magnesium plays important roles in the structure and the function of the human body, as it is involved in more than 300 essential metabolic reactions. **Foods: Brown rice, beans and peas, almonds, bananas, dark greens.**

Iron: Iron is essential for metabolism, blood health and immune system function. It is important to consume a wide variety of iron-rich foods on a daily basis, **including legumes, especially chickpeas, adzuki beans, lentils and kidney beans; nuts and seeds such as cashews, almonds, pumpkin seeds, sunflower seeds, and tahini (sesame); whole grains such as quinoa; fruits like dates, prunes, raisins, and dried fruits; and black strap molasses.**

*__Floradix Iron__ supplement is very good. A liquid formula with herbs and vitamins, it is easily absorbed and does not usually cause constipation.

Zinc: Zinc is essential for growth, cell structure and immunity. It appears to be vital in male reproduction and sexual function. **Foods: Cashews, almonds, beans, veggies.**

Trace Minerals: Elements required in small amounts by living organisms for normal growth. These include boron, chromium, cobalt, copper, iodine, manganese, molybdenum, phosphorus, potassium, and selenium. **Foods: Leafy greens, legumes, nuts/seeds, whole grains, and fruits like bananas, prunes and raisins.**

The Government Recommended Daily Allowances (RDA) for vitamins and minerals can be found at http://fnic.nal.usda.gov. You will find that eating real foods will provide you with adequate nutrients.

5. Fiber:

You have quite an extensive digestive tract. Your intestines are long by design so your body can extract the nutrients out of the food you have eaten and absorb them into your system. Fiber is essential, as it promotes bowel health and helps rid the body of toxins. In other words, fiber keeps you "regular," which helps decrease your risk of hemorrhoids, varicose veins, cancers, diabetes and constipation. **Foods: Just about every plant-based food contains fiber. Grains, beans, nuts/seeds, vegetables, and fruits. Yes, once again, nature knows best!**

6. Phytonutrients:

"Phyto" (meaning plant) nutrients are substances of plant origin that have significant health value. These compounds appear to provide added natural protection against diseases like cardiovascular disease, cancers and degeneration. They have anti-oxidant properties, which help with immunity, inflammation, growth, repair, and overall good health. The powerful Phytonutrients are 'freebies" that benefit your health just by eating. Fruits, vegetables, legumes, whole grains and nuts are rich in Phytonutrients. Nope, animal parts have no Phytonutrients. Once again, proof that nature loves you!

Vitamin Supplements? The debate rages on whether taking a supplement is helpful. In my clinical experience, I have recommended supplements to many patients with good results for a broad range of nutrient deficiency symptoms and chronic problems. Therefore, it may be a good idea to take a high-quality supplement, as life can be stressful and full of environmental toxins. It is important to use a pharmaceutical grade, high-quality multi-vitamin/mineral supplement. Be careful and do some research, as there are a bazillion supplement products on the market and even more sales people to sell you a "cure in a bottle."

If you are eating a nutrient rich diet like **The 16/21 Diet Solution**, you do not need to be on a $250.00 or more monthly supplement regime. A high-quality multi-vitamin should cost around $30-40 for a month's supply. Eating your nutrients through food is the best way to go, but a quality supplement might be good insurance, especially if you lead a stressful life. Supplements can help, but remember, **health does not come in a bottle!**

When looking at a supplement, ask for a copy of an independent analysis (called an assay) of the supplement ingredients you are thinking of buying. Any reputable company will have this analysis available to back their supplement. That is a good way to verify what you are buying. Also, look for **whole food extracted supplements**, as you do not want to take synthetic vitamins. They are not good for you. Defeats the purpose.

7. Water:

Water is very important for your health and essential for all of your processes. You must drink plenty of fresh water each day and it is best to drink throughout the day. Eating more fresh fruits, vegetables and fresh-squeezed juices each day can help improve nutrient and water intake. Another one of nature's diabolical plots to keep you healthy and vibrant.

Try not to drink large quantities of water at one time. You will get better utilization by drinking a smaller amount of water, more often. Drinking too large a quantity of water in a short time can cause you to feel "swishy" in your gut. Try drinking a small water cooler cup (about 4 ounces) twice per hour. That is 8 ounces of water per our in small amounts. After 8 hours you have taken on 64 ounces of water and with adequate hydration and no "swishy" feeling. You may find that you are urinating more frequently at first. This is normal, as your body is starting to process the increased water intake. As your system regulates to the increased intake of water, your frequency of urination will slow. Your system will enjoy working at an adequately hydrated level and your energy will also improve.

The Big Picture On Your Nutrient Needs:

- Remember, nature packed the nutrients you need within foods designed for you; vegetables, fruits, whole grains, beans, nuts, and seeds are your best sources for your nutrient needs.
- Consider taking a professional-grade vitamin/mineral supplement each day. I do believe vitamins are good insurance to "supplement" your needs, hence the name.

  B complex with B12 and folic acid, and A, C, D, E are a good idea.
- Do not rely on *any* supplement as a replacement for your nutrient intake. You must eat nutrient rich foods daily. There is no cure in a bottle!
- Many vitamins and minerals like vitamin D, calcium, vitamin B12, folic acid and iron are commonly fortified within pre-made items you can buy at the health food store, such as soy milks and cereals.
- Eat an abundant amount of nutrient-rich fruits, vegetables, legumes, whole grains and nuts each day. Be diverse and creative with your choices.
- Drink plenty of fresh clean water each day.
- Trust Nature; Eating foods designed for you is the key. So, eat, drink and be merry with high-powered foods!

CHAPTER 6

The 16/21 Diet Solution, "The Success Equation"

The 16/21 Diet Solution is your answer to the "*how do I eat healthier*" question. With **16/21**, you will find that you do not have to **count calories, deprive or starve yourself, or give up all your food vices to get the success you desire!**

My clinical experience treating thousands of patients has shown me many things about human nature. One thing I have discovered is that many people "need" their food vices at times. With as much that we all have to deal with in life, sometimes that rich, decadent chocolate cake or a grey goose and cranberry is *perfect* after a day in Purgatory.

It is abundantly clear that, at times, what we put in our mouth is our attempt to provide emotional and/or physical rescue for ourselves. Eating is such a big part of our comfort zone that it is the fiber that defines us as a nation and as individuals. My **16/21 Diet Solution** does not require you to abandon all your food vices. Absolutely not! That would be ridiculous, not to mention pure torture.

There is a way to eat for satisfaction and for health. Actually, eating healthy is satisfying and eating satisfactorlly is healthy. Even Willy Wonka would dig that line.

How The 16/21 Diet Solution Works:

There are 3 meals a day and 7 days in a week. Therefore you have 21 decisions per week regarding your meals. I like to look at meal choices as opportunities to enhance your health. You kill two stones with one bird. Eating which you need to do and enhancing your health which you want to do. Win-Win. How awesome is that!

My protocol and recipes help you make 16 meal choices that are very healthy, great tasting, quick and easy. You can take the other 5 meals per week and simply blow the doors off if you want to. If you have something you cannot live without, then **don't**! Go ahead, indulge and don't guilt trip yourself into oblivion. I have pointed out many of the items that are more dangerous to your health and reading my list may prompt you to want to throw this book into the trash. But wait a second. My diet protocol is designed for you to still be **you**. You will not have to join a cult, shave your head or change who you are. You enhance your health by enhancing your eating. Simple, easy and effective.

I have found that a patient's poor health is not coming from a handful of not-so-healthy meals each week. But be honest with yourself. If you are **not** eating **real foods** (see Chapter 2) often and you are eating a lot of junk each day, then your poor health is coming from more than 5 meals a week. Many people try to single out a couple things that are causing most of the trouble, but your body does not see it that way. Remember chronic inflammation? If you are eating toxic stuff on a regular basis, even in snack items, then you are skydiving with a tissue paper parachute.

Calorie Counting and Meal Proportions:

In my opinion, counting calories and meal proportion size is a ridiculous notion pawned off on the consumer. When eating nutriet rich-foods, you do not have to count calories or even watch your proportion sizes. **16/21** puts an abundance of nutrients in your body each day so the old paradigm of "watching what you eat" will hopefully finally die off for you.

The 16/21 Diet Solution allows you to **eat**. And eat like a real person. Yes, Americans over-consume. But we don't over-consume real food. We over-consume "junk food" products, man-made chemicals, and artificial flavors. That is how the counting calorie and proportion sizing came to be. All that stuff will make you fat, overweight, inflamed and **toxic**. Many "experts" tell you to eat less and restrict your calories. **That is insane**. Since the products you have been eating do not give you a solid nutrient intake anyway, **don't count it as eating!** Count it as what it is, "**junking out**!" But you still need to **eat real food** for health and life.

Do you wonder why you always seem hungry? That's **because you are hungry!** Eating meals made with real foods will give your body the nutrients it needs for energy and your body will start to work more efficiently. Your eating needs will be met and your body will stop banging on your insides for attention. Cutting calories and barely eating will put a strain on your body, your health, and everyone around you. Haven't you ever heard from a loved one or a co-worker, "Thank you, thank you, thank you," when you announce that you have quit the ridiculous "diet" you had been doing?

The 16/21 Diet Solution is not a radical fad "diet". I designed it for **real people** just like you. Listen, I was a full-time single dad of three teenagers. I was the maid, the cook, the shopper, the repairman, the mom and the dad. My kids gave me the acronym, "MAD" for mom and dad, though my suspicions are it had another definition they didn't tell me about. In my spare time, I treated patients and educated them to a healthier dietary path. So, take my word for it. **The 16/21 Diet Solution** recipes are easy, healthy, great tasting, and even the kids will love them.

In my design, I utilize foods that are nutrient-packed with full-spectrum flavor and have you eating them throughout your day. I am sure you heard of most all of the foods that are in my recipes, but you may not have incorporated them into your daily eating habits. At first it may feel scary, but after giving your body solid nutrients for about two weeks, you will start to see the amazing abilities your body has regarding healing and working more efficiently. You will see when you get to the menu plan (page 55) that you will be able to eat a good quantity of real food, feel great, and not be wishing you didn't eat so much. I am not advising for you to over-eat, but that is the beauty of eating foods designed for your physiology. Your body will help regulate your intake needs. When your nutrient uptake is satisfied your body is satisfied and happy!

The Big Idea approach to 16/21:

- **The 16/21 Diet Solution is an easy, real world approach.**
- **You will enjoy the 16 meals per week, as they are easy to make, taste great and give you the energy you need.**
- **You can also enjoy the 5 meals you can do whatever with *no guilt*. We don't do guilt, drama or dogma!**
- **Of course, if you would like to hit 21/21 then go right ahead.**
- **If you don't hit 16 out of 21 right away, just keep trying.**
- **You can do it.**

Your Perfect Diet Design Plan:

Let's put **The 16/21 Diet Solution** to work for you. I recommend you follow the 2-week menu plan to help you get comfortable with some new concepts and techniques. Drink plenty of fresh water throughout the day. I have intentionally left out desserts. I have included many in the recipe section, but I want you to experience this food transformation with the focus on the meals. If you are craving a dessert, try a piece of fruit or make one of the smoothies. Also, if you have a known allergy to something in one of the recipes, then omit that recipe and change it out for a different recipe choice. Each recipe provides a large amount so you can use leftover portions easily. Meal prep is quick and easy. Eat greens daily. They pack power!

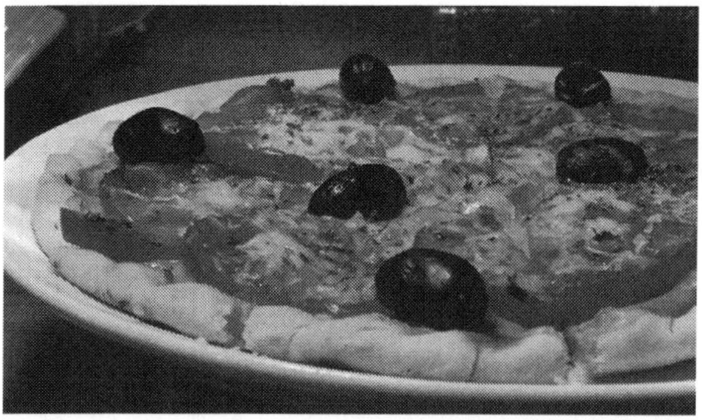

True Veggie Pizza (See www.docemerson.com for additional recipes.)

Note: The page number for each recipe is designate by ( )

WEEK 1:

Day 1

Breakfast: Green Power Smoothie (95), 16-ounce glass

Snack: Left over Green Power Smoothie

Lunch: All Star Salad (103) with Anti-Inflammatory Dressing (101)

Snack: Himalayan salted raw almonds, 2-3 handfuls

Dinner: Pesto Guarendo (112) toss with whole grain pasta, with mixed green salad + choice of dressings (101) (Make several of the dressings at one time and they will keep all week in airtight containers.)

Day 2

Breakfast: Black Pepper Grits (133) with whole grain toast and avocado as spread.

Snack: Organic Raw Food Bar (135)

Lunch: Avo-Cucumber Salad (104)

Snack: Raw Organic cashews, 2-3 handfuls

Dinner: Wrap-O-Meal (114) (Make several and use one on Day 3)

Day 3

Breakfast: Orange Juice Sunrise (97), 16-ounce glass

Snack: Organic Raw Food Bar (135)

Lunch: Left over Wrap-O-Meal

Snack: Raw Organic Fruit

Dinner: Lasagna (125) with mixed green salad

Day 4

Breakfast: Bananacado Smoothie (96), 16-ounce glass

Snack: Left over Bananacado Smoothie

Lunch: Left over Lasagna from dinner from Day 3

Snack: Raw Organic Cashews, 2-3 handfuls

Dinner: Miles' Famous Enchiladas (120) with mixed green salad

Day 5

Breakfast: Quick Power Cereal (132)

Snack: 1 sliced Organic Apple

Lunch: # 1 of 5 of open choice, otherwise known as "whatever"

Snack: Raw Organic Almonds or Cashews, 2-3 handfuls

Dinner: Jack Talk Thai (cooked version) (117) with Kale / Wakame Salad (105)

Day 6

Breakfast: Raisin-Berry Bran Cereal (133)

Snack: Raw Organic Fruit

Lunch: Avo-Delight (108) with Flax Crackers (135)

Snack: Raw Organic Cashews, 2-3 handfuls

Dinner: Raw Avochini Soup (109) with mixed green salad

(Prepare Stuffed Red Peppers (118) for Day 7)

Day 7

Breakfast: Berry Nut Smoothie (96), 16-ounce glass

Snack: Raw Organic Fruit

Lunch: 1-2 Stuffed Red Peppers (118)

Snack: Raw Organic Fruit

Dinner: Derek's Tofu Scramble (134) with whole grain toast and avocado spread

WEEK 2:

Day 8

Breakfast: Breakfast Burritos (134) with leftover Derek's Tofu Scramble

Snack: Organic Raw Food Bar (135)

Lunch: # 2 of 5 of open choice

Snack: Raw Organic Almonds soaked in Nama Shoyu, 2-3 handfuls

Dinner: Roma-Basil Sauce (113) with whole grain pasta and mixed green salad

Day 9

Breakfast: Green Power Smoothie (95), 16-ounce glass

Snack: Leftover Green Power Smoothie

Lunch: Meatless Meat Sandwich (130) with mixed green salad

Snack: Raw Organic Fruit

Dinner: Raw Caliente Soup (110) with Flax Crackers (135)

Day 10

Breakfast: Whole Grain Pancakes (131)

Snack: Raw Organic Fruit

Lunch: Rosemary Artichoke Hummus (107) with Organic Baby Carrots

Snack: Primal Strip (135)

Dinner: La Vita E'Buona (119) with raw veggie pasta and mixed green salad

Day 11

Breakfast: Coconut Almond Smoothie (97), 16-ounce glass

Snack: Leftover Coconut Almond Smoothie

Lunch: Awesome Pita Pockets (127) with mixed green salad

Snack: Raw Organic Baby Carrots

Dinner: # 3 of 5 of open choice

(Make Weight Loss Wraps (123) for Day 12.)

Day 12

Breakfast: Quick Power Cereal (132)

Snack: Raw Organic Fruit

Lunch: 3-4 Weight Loss Wraps (123)

Snack: Raw Veggies with Olive Oil, Balsamic Vinegar blend

Dinner: Shiitake Mushroom Soup (110) with mixed green salad

Day 13

Breakfast: Banango Smoothie (95), 16-ounce glass

Snack: Organic Raw Food Bar (135) or leftover Shiitake soup if available

Lunch: # 4 of 5 open choice

Snack: Primal Strip (135)

Dinner: Gabriela's Garlic Mashed Potatoes (123) with Kale / Wakame Salad (105)

Day 14

Breakfast: French Toast (131)

Snack: Raw Organic Fruit

Lunch: # 5 of 5 of open choice

Snack: Primal Strip (135)

Dinner: The Non-Believers Alfredo (121) with mixed green salad

Clinical Note:

Some patients have reported when they eat certain grains or grain products, they have a "heavy" feeling or feel bloated. My **16/21 Diet Solution** is designed to help you eliminate highly processed, refined products and eat real food more often. Not every ingredient used or suggested will work for everyone. If you have a known allergy, then substitute it for a different item. There are many substitution selections possible.
That is the beauty of plant-based foods. Be creative and I highly recommend for you to infuse more leafy greens, yellow veggies and raw fruits into your meals on a daily basis.
The more "power house" plant-based foods you eat, the better.

CHAPTER 7

Let's Go Shopping

When making changes to your diet, shopping healthier can be a little intimidating at first. It is actually easier than you may think, but takes a little getting used to. In this chapter, I have outlined what kind of foods to buy, where to get them and tools you will need. For years, I have taken patients on "field trips" to local markets, Whole Foods, Trader Joe's and even my own kitchen to learn more about healthy eating. It just takes a little getting used to. Kind of like life in general.

Proper Kitchen equipment and tools are very important to your diet and health. Since you are going to be more health conscious by eating better, buying organic food and preparing recipes, it is just as important NOT to use cheap, toxic kitchen tools that can sink the ship. Quality tools are an investment in your health and are invaluable to your cooking experience.

Kitchen Tools: The Must Haves

- ❑ **Blender:** Ideally, commercial grade. I personally use the *K-Tech Blender*. It can take a beating and blend up dang near everything. *Vita-Mix* is another good blender.
- ❑ **Food Processor:** The commercial grade *Cuisinart* is a good processor; *Kitchen Aid* makes a good one, too. Make sure it is high capacity for volume and power. 12-14 cups capacity.
- ❑ **Juicer:** There are many juicers available. I like The *Jack LaLanne* brand. Champion and Green Star are also good juicers.

- ❑ **Knives:** I use 3 kitchen knives and that is about all I use.
  - ❑ **A cleaver**
  - ❑ **A chef's knife**
  - ❑ **A paring knife or short knife**

  Note: It is important to keep your knives sharp. A sharp knife is a safer knife.
- ❑ **Cutting board:** I prefer a non-wood board as it is easier to clean, about 8 X 12 inches; the bigger the better.
- ❑ **Coffee grinder:** An electric coffee grinder is a nice tool for grinding spices and seeds. Good for flax meal from flax seeds. Making flax meal yourself is economical and easy.
- ❑ **Pots and pans:** It is best to cook with stainless steel cookware. You should avoid non-stick cookware, as the Teflon will come off over time and is not the best thing for your health. *All-Clad* makes good stainless steel cookware and is located in many stores like *Macy's*, etc. They can be an initial expensive investment, but I have a few *All-Clad* pans older than my teenagers. *Costco* carries a less expensive version of stainless steel cookware as well. You don't need toxic non-stick spray either. Pans will season with normal use, no problem. Medium, large and extra large saucepans, stock pots and fry pans.
- ❑ **Cast iron skillet:** A large cast iron skillet is a great old world pan that can help add iron to your diet through cooking.
- ❑ **Rice cooker:** This is a must. This will make your life easier and your rice will come out perfect. You can cook a wide variety of whole grain rice, wild rice and even quinoa in a rice cooker. www.LotusFoods.com sells a great 12-cup stainless steel cooker for around $80 plus shipping. Also comes with a steamer insert so you can steam veggies al dente toward the end of the cooking cycle.
- ❑ **Measuring cups:** Buy 3 Pyrex glass cups: a 4-cup, 2-cup and 1-cup size.
- ❑ **Measuring spoons:** Stainless steel set will last a lifetime.

- ❑ **Utensils:** Keep a variety of stainless steel items handy:
  - ❑ **Large kitchen spoon**
  - ❑ **Large ladle**
  - ❑ **Tongs**
  - ❑ **Large and small spatula**
  - ❑ **Large pasta fork**
  - ❑ **Various size stainless strainers and a big colander**
  - ❑ **Hand-held julienne** (cutting veggies into strips)
- ❑ **Can opener:** A good sturdy hand-held works fine.
- ❑ **Garlic press:** Hand-held press, you will need one.
- ❑ **Cheese grater:** Box style is more stable than hand-held.
- ❑ **Pepper grinder:** Fresh crushed pepper will give your recipes a wonderful flavor that pre-ground pepper just can't provide.
- ❑ **Mixing bowls:** Essential for marinating and mixing items together during recipe building. Use stainless steel, glass, *Earthenware*. Small, medium, large and extra large.
- ❑ **Baking sheets:** Commercial grade cookie sheets are tough and will last a long time. Avoid the non-stick ones.
- ❑ **Baking dish:** For making enchiladas and casseroles, *Pyrex Glassware* makes very good baking dishes.
- ❑ **Storage containers:** A must for storing leftovers, soaked nuts and taking food with you when you are out. Must be sealable. *Sam's Club* or *Costco*.
- ❑ **Apple corer/wedger:** A great tool that quickly cores an apple and cuts it into wedges. Great for taking cut apples to work/ school in zip-lock bag. *OXO* makes a good one.
- ❑ **Mango pitter:** Like the apple corer, just bigger. Will change your thoughts about using mangos, as it is easy and awesome. The mango seed is an odd shape and can be a pain to work with but this tool is nearly foolproof. *OXO* brand is good.

- ❑ **www.williams-sonoma.com** They have most everything you need. Also, your local kitchen supply stores can be helpful. Look at the outlet malls, too.
- ❑ **Nut milk bag:** A small nylon bag with fine mesh to strain pulp from nut milks used in some of our recipes.

Other tools available: (not necessary, but helpful)

- ❑ **Mandolin:** For cutting a variety of veggies and fruits in creative shapes. *OXO* makes a good not so expensive one.
- ❑ **Dehydrator:** This is a machine that dehydrates fruits and veggies at a low temp to maximize nutrients. Great for making flax "crackers," pizza crusts and your own dried fruits and nuts. Once you start eating these items, you will never want a greasy chip again. I think *Excalibur's* are the best ones made. www.excaliburdehydrator.com
- ❑ **Garlic peeler:** Actually peels cloves for you in a couple seconds, which makes pressing garlic way easier.
- ❑ **Avocado slicer:** Creates uniform avocado slices for beautiful presentation.
- ❑ **Citrus juicer:** A glass one is nice to have, but the old fashion squeeze the tar out of it with your hand technique works too.

Foods:

Organic vs. Conventional?:

I am a firm believer in buying and eating organically grown foods as much as possible. The certification and labeling has become far more reliable than in the past. I recommend you look for certified organic foods as a first choice. Conventionally grown foods have been grown using pesticides and synthetic chemicals. Obviously, eating any kind of toxic chemicals is not a good idea, but there are times when organic is either not available or out of season, especially while eating out or traveling. You should also look to your local farmers markets. Many local farmers grow their crops without pesticides or chemicals, but they have not gone through the expensive certification process to become “Certified Organic.” For many local farmers to be certified is not cost-effective. Get to know these hard-working farmers. You will probably find they are wonderful people and have a wealth of knowledge for what they grow, with high ethical standards for their craft.

Is organic more expensive? In some cases, yes. But is saving a little money by eating toxins and poisons a good idea? Y**our health should be worth the investment. Go natural and go organic as often as you can.**

Genetic Modified Organisms (GMO’s):

I recommend you do not eat foods that have been genetically modified. GMO foods are making their way into **everything**. It is estimated 80% of all processed foods contain GMO’s. Nearly all livestock in the USA are fed GMO feed. This ends up in you when you eat those animal parts. Farm raised salmon are fed GMO corn and soy meal. Not actually their native food supply. I recommend everyone should find out all they can about GMO’s and their dangers. This book is about eating healthier. One can write an entire book on the dangers of GMO’s. In fact, there are several good ones out there. Briefly stated, the manipulation behind GMO’s is quite scary. Natural occurring compounds (fruits & vegetables) cannot be patented, since they are naturally occurring. However, GMO’s have been “altered” and are now patented products but still called foods.

But in reality, these "foods" have been manipulated and are no longer natural, not even close. The companies that make GMO's have gone to lengths to get our greedy little law makers to allow items made with GMO's to avoid labeling. There is **no label requirement** for GMO products in the USA. Like, WTF? Are you kidding me? Unproven genetic manipulated junk in our food supply and it doesn't even get a label, a disclaimer or a warning sign? Yep! Welcome to Washington. Due to this cute little political side-step, you are eating GMO's everyday and don't even know it. Most other countries around the world require mandatory labeling. However, the good news, here in the US, most conscious health food suppliers label their item Non-GMO. Read labels. A reputable natural food company will never use GMO's. There are good sites to learn more about GMO's, including www.saynotogmos.org.

Hierarchy of Nutrient Composition in Foods:

If there ever was to be a ranking system of the best foods to eat, I think it should be based on the amount of nutrients and where it ranks within nature. Nutrient rich foods are what your body needs for good health.

You will see that I use organic canned and organic frozen foods in some recipes. Hey, this is the real world and your time can be short. Besides, it is a big jump up in nutrients compared to heavily refined, processed junk items. So, don't worry using some foods that are minimally helped along by good health-conscious companies. Once again, avoid GMO's.

The 16/21 Diet Solution Nutrient Food Choice Ranking:

1. **Organic Fresh Raw Fruits, Vegetables, Nuts, Seeds, & Sprouts.** You cannot get more high-powered than in the **raw**. To me, there is no argument needed. Raw plant-based foods are the pinnacle. The more often you can eat raw, the better. **16/21** has a large selection of raw recipes and meals that will surprisingly blow your mind…in a good way.
2. **Organic Whole Grains, Legumes, Veggies and Fruits (cooked):** Veggies should be lightly steamed or sautéed, always al dente to retain as much nutrients as possible. Sorry mom, boiling the broccoli to death makes it nearly useless. But I do love you… ☺
3. **Organic Canned or Organic Frozen Fruits, Veggies, Beans, etc.:** Yes there can be an argument for canned foods being less nutrient-rich than fresh. However, since eating healthier has allowed more conscious companies to be profitable and still in business, you can now buy organic canned veggies, beans and fruit that have been minimally processed. These are usually never refined, just ready for you to use. These items have come light-years compared to the 1960's and 70's canned foods. *Eden Foods* is a wonderful company that makes very good organic food items.
4. **Organic Boxed or Pre-Made Organic Frozen or Cooler items:** There are some good items that do come in a box on the shelf or are found in the freezer/fridge section of the natural food store. For instance *Amy's Kitchen* makes very good frozen items that make great quick snacks or even a meal. These are a far cry improvement from the nutrient lacking TV dinners and "hamburger helper" type meals we had when we were kids.
5. **When in doubt:** When you are considering if something is good for you or not, think of the **16/21** ranking system. If it does not fall into #1-4, you may want to avoid it altogether. Of course you can use one of your 5 "blow it" meals to consume something you know is not good for you, but you want it anyway.

Please read the list of ingredients to avoid in Appendix C in the back of the book, as these items are known to cause problems in humans and it is best to avoid them.

The Shopping list is designed to help you get comfortable with finding and identifying foods at the natural food stores. You do not need to buy everything at once. Just spend some time getting to know your store and the items listed. Visit local natural food markets, these good people are usually willing to order or carry a product/food item you like if you don't see it in their store. Similar to local farmers, these store owners are in the business of health food for a reason, they believe in eating healthier and sharing the idea with everyone. We are now ready to get familiar with these wonderful life enhancing foods. So:

Ready, Set, Shop!

Oils:

Once again, first and foremost **eliminate** harmful **trans fats** (hydrogenated vegetable oils) from your diet. These oils are highly **toxic** to your health. They are in most processed "food" products.

Buy **organic, unrefined, expeller-pressed oils** to ensure maximum purity, flavor and nutrition whenever possible. Choosing organic oils can also minimize your exposure to pesticides. Many pesticides are fat-soluble (remember, oil is a fat) and are found in many conventional oils.

Understanding Oils in the Kitchen:

Natural, expeller pressed plant oils have a good nutrient composition so when you use oils for nutrients, eat them **raw, just as they are, as oils**.

For cooking, remember you are facilitating heat to the foods through the oil. But heating the oil does decrease the natural nutrient levels. A lot of oil is not needed. A little bit goes a long way. When cooking with oils, it is **important** to know heating the particular oil beyond its **smoke point** is not good—in fact, it can be **toxic**. The smoke point is the temperature at which the oil begins to smoke, generating toxic fumes and creating harmful free-radicals in the oil. If you do smoke the oil by accident, always discard the oil along with any food in contact with the burned oil and start over. Most natural oil companies label the suggested temperatures for cooking on the bottle. Read the label of a particular oil to determine its smoke point and never heat the oil higher than this temperature. There are different oils for low, medium and high heats (see table below). In general, refined oils will have a higher smoke point than unrefined oils. Health conscious oil companies may refine the oil a touch for stability, but their process does not use caustic chemicals and they **are not** trans fats. There are several wonderful companies listed in Appendix B: Company List at the back of this book.

Unrefined oil is pressed and bottled and that's it. This old-world, low-tech, method helps retain the oils original nutrient content, flavor and color. They are truly the best. Raw, unrefined oils do not have a long shelf life, but they will give you great flavor and high nutrients. Raw, unrefined oils are not only healthy for you, but they also add full-bodied flavor to dishes, sauces, dressings, marinades, and dipping.

Healthy Oils:

Try all of these oils raw, not heated, for added taste, nutrients, and a touch of nirvana. Buy in smaller amounts for freshness.

- Almond Oil
- Avocado Oil
- Borage Oil
- Apricot Oil
- Coconut Oil
- Flaxseed Oil
- Hazelnut Oil
- Hempseed Oil
- Macadamia Nut Oil
- Olive Oil
- Palm Oil
- Peanut Oil
- Pecan Oil
- Sesame Oil
- Walnut Oil

I like to use many of the above oils on whole grain toasts, dips for veggies and all salad dressings. Great taste and much healthier for you.

Heat and light are especially harmful to oils, so they should be kept in the refrigerator. The oil may cloud some in the fridge but it does not affect quality or benefits of the oil. Do not store oils near your stove, as excessive heat from the stove or oven can ruin the oils.

As stated before, it is important to use the correct oil at the correct temperature when cooking and baking. Using the correct oil will add to the quality of the recipe and the overall taste. Many good recipes have been ruined by using the incorrect temperature for the oil used.

Best Oils for Specific Cooking Temperatures:

Best for Baking:

- Coconut oil
- Palm oil
- Safflower oil
- Sunflower oil

Best for Low Heats:

- Most every oil (except hempseed)

Best for Medium Heats & Sautéing:

- Coconut oil
- Hazelnut oil
- Macadamia nut oil
- Pecan oil
- Safflower oil (high oleic)
- Sesame oil
- Sunflower oil (high oleic)
- Walnut oil

Best for High Heat & Frying:

- Almond oil
- Avocado oil
- Apricot oil
- Sesame oil
- Safflower oil (high oleic)
- Sunflower oil (high oleic)
- Coconut oil

Note: Hempseed oil is wonderful for health, but should never be heated! It is too fragile to be used with heat. Raw only. ☺

Note on cooking with olive oil:

Olive oil is indeed good for you; however, I have read many times the suggestion of frying or high-heat cooking with olive oil for good health.

Olive oil is a medium to low-heat oil, and low-heat sautéing. Higher temps ruin the oil and negate the benefits you desire.

One of my favorites: *Bariani Olive Oil*. Stone-crushed, old-school olive oil is very good, especially in the raw. www.barianioliveoil.com

Organic Nuts, Seeds and Their Butters:

Organic raw nuts and seeds are good sources of essential fatty acids, anti-oxidants, protein and trace minerals. A quality source of good fats as they have no trans-fats and no cholesterol. They have been thrown under the "too high in fat" bus, but the wonderful health benefits are putting a lot of old myths to rest. Nuts and seeds make for a healthier snack than the standard junk food items.

Try not to use the standard roasted nuts as they are usually roasted in poor quality oils. Once you start eating raw nuts and seeds you will understand how wonderful they are and how good you feel eating them. **Unless you have a known allergy, try them all. Buy organic** whenever possible:

- Almonds & Almond butter
- Brazil Nuts
- Cashews & Cashew Butter
- Chestnuts
- Flax Seed
- Hazelnuts & Hazelnut Butter
- Hemp Seeds and Hemp Butter
- Macadamia Nuts & Macadamia Butter
- Peanuts & Peanut Butter
- Pecans
- Pine Nuts
- Pistachios
- Pumpkin Seeds
- Sesame Seeds (Tahini is the Butter)
- Sunflower Seeds & Sunflower Seed Butter
- Walnuts and Walnut Butter

Remember To Soak Your Nuts: ☺

For nuts, seeds and butters, buying and eating them raw will give you the highest nutrient base. With the exception of Brazil, hazelnuts and macadamias, you **should soak** raw nuts and seeds to make their nutrients more bio-available and easier to digest. Nuts have a natural enzyme-inhibitor, which protects them in the wild, but makes them a little harder to digest. Generally, nuts should be soaked for about 8 hours. For walnuts and pecans, 2 hours is sufficient. It is easy to soak the nuts overnight. Just put them in a bowl and cover the nuts with fresh water before you go to bed. In the morning, simply rinse them well with fresh water in a strainer, pat them dry with a paper towel, and then store in airtight container and put back in fridge until you are ready to use them. Do not keep or use the water the nuts were soaking in; discard down the drain. They will keep for a few days in the fridge in an airtight container, and are ready to use for the multitude of creations nuts can provide. Once again, avoid using nuts roasted with highly processed conventional oils.

You can eat nuts raw, seasoned with Himalayan salt, and use in many recipes for great flavor and added nutrients. For a nice treat, you can soak almonds, sunflower seeds, cashews, etc. in Nama Shoyu soy sauce for 1 hour. Pour off soy sauce, place in zip-lock bag with salt, shake, and take with you for a great travel snack.

Roasted Nuts and Seeds (Homemade version)

Make your own: Place nuts or seeds on a baking sheet, sprinkle with Himalayan salt, and heat in the oven at 375° F for 3-5 minutes. No additional oil needed.

Keep an eye on them, as nuts don't have a lot of water in them and can burn quickly. Been there done that!

Whole Grains and Whole Grain Flours:

Eating whole grains and using whole grain flours in your cooking recipes will provide you with nutrients and fiber. They will also fill the void of empty nutrient, high calorie products you have been eating that are "refined" grains and flours. Remember the carb confusion:
refined = junk; whole grains = nutrients.

The nutrient rich part of the grain is called the kernel and it has three layers. The outside is the **bran**, the middle is the **germ**, and the inner core is the **endosperm**. The bran and germ are rich in B-vitamins, minerals and fiber. In the refining process, whole grains are stripped of the bran and germ, destroying the majority of the grain's nutrients and flavor. Refining companies sell "enriched' white flour products which have been processed with harsh chemicals. A handful of vitamins are added, but it can never duplicate nature's original design. Remember, "enriched" is now a product, not a food.

Whole grains have a wonderful balance of complex carbohydrates, protein, and are naturally low in fat. They can be found in packages or in the bulk section of the store. Follow the cooking instructions on the package or many stores have pre-printed instructions you can take home.

NG= non-gluten

- Amaranth – **NG**
- Barley, Pearled and Flakes
- Buckwheat Flour – **NG**
- Corn Grits (polenta) – **NG**
- Cornmeal, Blue/Yellow – **NG**
- Couscous
- Kamut, Whole Grain and Flakes
- Millet – **NG**
- Popcorn – **NG**
- Quinoa – **NG**
- Rolled Oats
- Rye

- Soy Flour – **NG**
- Spelt and Spelt Flakes
- Steel Cut Oats
- Wheat: Bulgur, Cracked, Flakes
- Whole Wheat Flours: Whole wheat, Durum and Pastry

My guess is you probably don't have time to make your own whole grain pastas every week, so instead of buying "refined" inflammation creating white pastas, buy Organic whole grain ones. They are delicious and much better for you.

Whole Grain Pastas:

Try to use organic whole grain pastas only. Whole grain pastas are wonderfully diverse in flavor and textures, and high in nutrients.

- **Corn Pasta:** A nutty-corn taste, medium dense pasta. This pasta is a good alternative to whole wheat pastas.
- **Durum Semolina Pasta:** A nice whole-wheat pasta that is versatile to use.
- **Japanese Pastas:** Whole grain, highly nutritious and great tasting. Great for soups, veggie stir-fry's or in the usual pasta dishes.
  - **Udons:** A whole wheat pleasant tasting pasta.
  - **Soba:** A buckwheat pasta, great tasting and high in nutrients.
  - **Lomein:** A whole-wheat lighter flavored noodle pasta.
- **Orzo (wheat):** It is rice shaped but made from hard wheat semolina.
- **Jerusalem Artichoke Pasta:** Has slightly lower carbohydrate content and a mild, pleasant flavor.
- **Kamut:** Pasta that is high-gluten, high-protein content, whole-grain that has a rich, buttery flavor.
- **Spelt:** Made from a variety of wheat that many people find more easily digested than durum wheat.
- **Sesame-Rice Pasta:** Consists of 80% durum wheat, 10% brown rice and 10% sesame flour. Tends to be a little higher in protein than other pastas.

- **Quinoa:** An ancient grain used by the Incas, is a wonderful light and fluffy, highly nutritious grain. Cooks easily in a rice cooker—simple, easy and awesome.
- **Sprouted Wheat Pasta:** Made with a combination of sprouted grains, such as wheat, barley, millet, lentils and soy.

Organic Rices:

Rice is one of the most versatile food items to have on hand. It can be used in nearly any recipe, is easily digested, and it will provide you with a lot of nutrients. Minimize the use of white rice in your diet.

- **Brown Rice:** Comes in **short, long and basmati grains**. Brown rice should be a staple in your kitchen and diet. Very versatile and highly nutritious. (I like *Lundberg* rice: www.lundberg.com)
- **Forbidden Black:** Deep purple-black in color and looks intense, but this rice is full of fragrant aromas, a nutty taste, with high nutritional value.
- **Kalijira:** A Tender and sweet rice, highly aromatic, like Basmati.
- **Bhutanese Red:** Grown at 8,000 feet in the Himalayan Kingdom of Bhutan, this premium heirloom rice contains trace minerals, has a nutty/earthy flavor, soft texture and beautiful red russet color.
- **Black Japonica:** A blend of 25% black short-grain japonica and 75% medium-grain mahogany-red rice. Chewy, but tender with a full flavor that's good in stuffing or rice salads.
- **Jade Pearl:** Infused with bamboo extract, made from the Moso species of bamboo that grows in the virgin highland forest of south central China. Gives this medium grain rice the aroma of a bamboo forest, a light vanilla taste, and an explosion of health-giving nutrients. www.LotusFoods.com
- **Wild Rice:** A hearty flavored rice, high in protein (10 grams/cup). Great for a change of rice and winter holiday meals.

A rice cooker (stainless steel insert) is invaluable. You can cook many grains in a rice cooker with good success. Make up 10-12 cups at one time and store in airtight container to use all week in recipes.

Organic Legumes (Beans):

Beans are versatile, good sources of protein, and are stocked full of many vitamins and minerals. They can be utilized raw/sprouted (highest nutrient value), cooked at home, or using organic canned is fine, too.

- **Adzuki**
- **Black**
- **Black-Eyed Peas**
- **Cannellini**
- **Chickpeas**
- **Fava**
- **Great Northern**
- **Lentils (all varieties)**
- **Lima (Butter)**
- **Mung**
- **Navy**
- **Peas, Split Peas**
- **Pinto**
- **Red Kidney**
- **Soy**

Cooked beans can give you a little gas. Cooking beans with Kombu can help reduce this phenomenon. Kombu is a sea vegetable that works well in helping to "de-gas" your cooking beans. Add a two-inch strip per one cup of dried beans during cooking. Also, pre-cooked organic canned beans are available. www.edenfoods.com makes ready-made canned Organic beans with Kombu added and are delicious.

Organic Vegetables:

Can be eaten raw, juiced, lightly steamed, sautéed, or baked. Use organic fresh, organic frozen, organic canned, or organic dehydrated. It is important to buy organic whenever possible. It is worth the money.

Vegetables and fruits are high in nutrients, antioxidants, fiber, and low in calories. In my program, we don't count calories. Why? If you compare a piece of steak that has 500 calories to 500 calories of vegetables, you will see the steak portion is very small, leaving you hungry, while the vegetable portion is abundant in amount, nutrients and satisfaction to your hunger. With vegetables, particularly leafy greens, the more you eat, the more weight you will lose and the more energy you will gain.

Dark Leafy Greens: (Natures power-packed plants)

- **Arugula:** Dark green, jagged leaves with a hearty, peppery flavor and a delicate texture. Great raw and mixes well with other greens. Is great in salads and sandwiches.
- **Beet Greens:** Bright green leaves offset by red stems and veins; often available bunched with their roots (beets). Mild greens, slightly sweet, tender leaves.
- **Bok Choy:** Soft, dark green leaves and long, thick white stalks with a sweet, mild flavor. Can be added to salads and soups, or lightly steamed.
- **Collards:** Big, round, flat gray-green leaves that encircle thick stalks. Their seemingly tough leaves become nicely tender after cooking, but can still be used raw as a wrap. Raw, steam or sauté.
- **Dandelion Greens:** Slightly bitter flavored green, notched leaves. Dandelion greens are wonderful raw or sautéed.
- **Endive:** Also called chicory, it has curly, frilly, coarse leaves, dark green edges, and pale yellow stems.
- **Kale:** Deep dark bluish-green, finely curled. Kale is delicious raw, added to vegetable soups, steamed or sautéed.

- **Spinach:** Tender, sweet green leaves. Best tasting eaten raw; versatile too, as you can add to smoothies, soups or sautéed.
- **Swiss Chard:** Red and green chard is common. Rainbow chard with pink, yellow and orange stems is a really good, too, but harder to find. Among the most versatile greens, chard can be prepared in numerous ways: raw, sautéed, in soups or rice dishes.
- **Turnip Greens:** Sharply but agreeably bitter, turnip greens, like beet greens, are often available with their roots.
- **Lettuces:** Butter, Green Leaf, Red Leaf, Romaine, Mesclun

Additional Wonderful Vegetables:

- **Artichokes:** Whole or the hearts packed in fresh water. Contains healthy amounts of minerals like calcium, magnesium and iron. They also contain several B vitamins and lots of lutein/zeaxanthins.
- **Asparagus:** Lightly steamed, good source of vitamins, minerals and fiber.
- **Beets:** Baby, Blood, and Golden. High in folate and good detoxifier.
- **Brussels Sprouts:** Contain cancer-fighting compounds sulforaphane and indole-3 carbinol; vitamin C, vitamin A and lutein.
- **Broccoli:** Green and Purple; called super food for the many health benefits and anti-cancer properties.
- **Cauliflower:** White, Yellow, Purple. Highly recommended as a cancer fighter, too.
- **Cabbages:** Red, Purple, Green. Contain glucosinolates, which may help to prevent cancer.
- **Carrots:** Large, Medium and Baby. Contain large amount of vitamin A and falcarinol, which may prevent cancer.
- **Celery:** Good for digestion as a juice or eaten raw.
- **Cucumbers**: Good source of vitamins A and C, and minerals. Good for digestion, especially prepared as fresh juice. Often used topically as beauty treatments for eyes. Place several slices in pitcher of ice water.
- **Eggplant:** Various shapes and sizes. High in antioxidants.
- **Garlic:** Good immune system booster and great flavor.

- **Green Beans:** Contain healthy amounts of calcium, vitamin C, beta Carotene, vitamin K and lutein.
- **Jicama:** Potato-like texture, use raw in salads, very nutritious.
- **Leeks:** Excellent source of vitamin A, beta carotene, lutein and folate.
- **Okra:** Traditionally, fried in the south, but even better raw.
- **Onions:** Red, Yellow, Green and Maui Sweet.
- **Peppers:** Green, Orange, Red, Yellow. Good source of vitamin A and vitamin C.
- **Potatoes:** Brown, Gold, Purple, Red.
- **Radish:** Red, Daikon, Long Scarlet.
- **Rhubarb:** Good source of magnesium, fiber, vitamin C, vitamin K, calcium, potassium and manganese.
- **Sprouts:** Alfalfa, Broccoli, Clover, Dill, Mung Bean, Radish, and Sunflower. Use raw in salads, sandwiches and juices. High in protein, vitamins A, C and K, niacin, thiamin, riboflavin, folate, pantothenic acid, iron, magnesium, phosphorus, zinc, copper, calcium and manganese.
- **Squash:** Acorn, Butternut, Pumpkin, Spaghetti, Yellow, Zucchini.
- **Sunchoke:** aka Jerusalem Artichoke, potato-like texture, best raw.
- **Tomatoes:** Beefsteak, Cherry, Heirloom, Roma, Sun-dried.
- **Turnips:** Blood cleanser. Good source of vitamin C, fiber and lutein.

Mushrooms:

Fungus among us: Use them raw, dried, sautéed, grilled and stuffed. Wash before use.

- **Chanterelles:** Golden color, delicate, wonderful taste.
- **Chicken of the Woods:** Bright yellow-orange, meaty texture, great as a meat substitute in recipes. Fools many meat eaters.
- **Creminis:** Are actually **baby portabella mushrooms** and easy to use.
- **Oysters:** Grayish-blue, mild flavor, sautés well.

- **Portabellas:** Add flavor to a sauté. Portabellas are wonderful grilled and used in sandwiches, burger style. They can be cut up and added to rice or pasta dishes. Portabellas are meaty, hearty and can also be stuffed.
- **Shiitakes:** Most versatile in my opinion, they have a wonderful woodsy flavor and chewy texture. Shiitakes are touted as a potent immune booster and cancer fighter.

Fruits:

Organic fresh, raw fruits are very important. They are stocked full of vitamins, minerals, Phytonutrients and water. They also help power you through the day much better than JUNK items. I recommend you eat fresh, organic, raw as much as possible. Organic raw frozen is fine, too. www.CascadianFarms.com is a good company for organic raw fruits in the freezer section of natural foods store.

- **Apples:** There are many different types of apples, including Ambrosia, Fuji, Gala, Golden, Granny Smith and Pippins. A good for source of fiber, vitamins and minerals.
- **Avocado:** Actually a fruit and very versatile and tasty, and contains good fats. Avocados are nutrient-dense and can be used for most anything.
- **Bananas:** Keep a couple in the freezer, as they work well for smoothies. Good source of vitamins B6 and C, potassium, manganese and fiber.
- **Berries:** Anti-oxidants and loaded with taste, eat them daily.
    - **Blueberries**
    - **Blackberries**
    - **Cranberries**
    - **Raspberries**
    - **Strawberries**
- **Cherries:** Bing, Brooks, Chelan, Lapin, Rainier.
- **Dates/Figs:** Very nutritious by themselves and dates make a good natural sweetener for recipes with added nutrients. Good source of B vitamins and iron.

- **Jackfruit:** Not easy to find, but good tasting, and high in manganese and vitamin C.
- **Kiwi:** An apple-strawberry flavor fruit, not just a bird or someone from New Zealand.
- **Lemons:** Several varieties, good for many recipes, like your ice water.
- **Limes:** Like lemons, versatile; but don't fruit beer, that's odd. ☺
- **Lychees:** A delicious, succulent fruit with a hard outer shell. Peel away the shell to find juicy, sweet inside with a center seed.
- **Mangos:** High in vitamins A, C and E, potassium and fiber.
- **Oranges:** All varieties, high in vitamins A and C.
- **Papayas:** Wonderful for digestion enzymes and other nutrients.
- **Pears:** Several varieties, good source of vitamin C, folic acid, and fiber.
- **Persimmons:** High in iron and vitamins A, B's, and C.
- **Pineapples:** Eating raw, fresh pineapple is very good for inflammation. Make fresh juice by removing the top, cutting fruit into strips and juice the strips, rind and all.
- **Raisins:** Flame, Golden, Thompson for iron and other minerals.
- **Star Fruit:** High in vitamins C and E. No peeling required, just cut across the fruit to reveal natural star shape.
- **Tangerines:** Sweet little fruit, high in vitamin C, and one of my favorite Led Zeppelin songs.

Dried fruits can make a great snack. Look for ones that do not have added sugar or sulfur. It makes no sense to eat a healthy dried fruit with added white refined sugar or toxic sulfur on it. If you have a dehydrator, you can make your own at home that are healthy and taste great.

Avocados are a great source of vitamins, minerals, protein, good fats, and essential fatty acids. You can use them in many ways. I use them as a condiment in sandwich making. Instead of high fat, inflammatory mayo, use the avocado as a spread. Use in fresh salads, dressing making, and smoothies.

Herbs (Fresh):

Culinary herbs are a great way to add anti-oxidants, phytonutrients and great flavor to your food. Many of these herbs are currently under clinical studies, as they suggest promising medicinal qualities. They have been used for thousands of years with good results. Imagine that...☺

- **Basil:** Antimicrobial and immune system stimulator.
- **Cilantro:** Antimicrobial, good for digestion and joint pains.
- **Dill:** Good for digestion by relieving intestinal gas. Improves bad breath, too.
- **Fennel:** High in anti-oxidants, blood cleanser.
- **Ginger:** Very good for digestion, can use in recipes, juicing and teas.
- **Lemon Grass:** Antibacterial, antifungal, used for insomnia and detoxification purposes.
- **Mint:** Sooths digestive tract, antifungal. Possibly helps allergies and asthma.
- **Oregano:** Antibacterial, antifungal, antiparasitic, Can be used in tablet form for colds and other viral infections.
- **Parsley:** Good for digestion, relieves intestinal gas.
- **Rosemary:** Antioxidant, antifungal, good for joint pains and digestion.
- **Thyme:** Antiparasitic, used as tea for relief of menstrual cramps and PMS.

Dried or Powder:

- **Bay leaves**
- **Black Peppercorn (to crush your own pepper)**
- **Cardamom**
- **Cayenne Powder**
- **Cinnamon Powder**
- **Cumin Powder**
- **Mustard Seed Powder**
- **Nutmeg Powder**
- **Onion Powder**
- **Oregano Dried**
- **Paprika Powder**
- **Red Chili Flakes**
- **Tarragon**
- **Turmeric Powder:** Helpful in reducing inflammation and pains; current studies as treatment for cancer, Alzheimer's and Parkinson's disease.

Salt:

Salt is essential for life; you actually cannot live without it. However, most people don't realize there are enormous differences between the standard, refined table and natural edible mineral salts.

Table salt is actually 97.5% sodium chloride and 2.5% chemicals, such as moisture absorbents and iodine. Dried at over 1,200° F, the excessive heat alters the natural chemical structure of the salt. Table salt is a "processed" item and one that should be avoided. Many doctors say not to eat table salt and I agree. Table salt is not good for you. It can offset your water balance, cause bloating, and leach the body of other nutrients. Natural mineral salts, are a better alternative for your body as they contain trace minerals and do not appear to cause health problems.

Salts I prefer:

- **Celtic Sea Salt:** This is a brand name and the company claims it to be an authentic, unprocessed, whole salt from one of the most pristine coastal regions of France. I honestly don't know if there is a pristine coastal region anywhere on the planet, but I do like Celtic salt, as I have used it for many years.
- **Himalayan Pink Crystal Salt:** This is my all time favorite salt to use raw and in meal prep. Pink in color, it is a tasty salt that brightens your meals with great flavor and added nutrients.

Dairy Substitutes:

For better health and a wonderful way to cut cholesterol and animal fat out of your diet is to use dairy substitutes. There are many delicious, versatile, nutritious food items found at natural food stores that make for a better choice than consuming bovine breast fluid (cow's milk).

- **Bean, Nut and Grain Milks:** The most commonly known is soy milk. However, there are several other milks that are delicious and **fortified** with vitamins and minerals and are good protein sources.
  - **Almond Milk**
  - **Hazelnut Milk**
  - **Coconut Milk**
  - **Oat Milk**
  - **Rice Milk**
- **Soy or Coconut Milk Yogurts:** Great tasting, fortified alternative to dairy based yogurts. No cholesterol.
- **Non-Dairy Cheese:** There are several dairy alternative choices. Some soy cheeses do contain casein or caseinate, which is a dairy milk protein and can be an allergen to many people. For a cheese alternative to contain milk protein defeats the purpose. I recommend, Vegan cheeses made by www.FollowYourHeart.com, as there is no animal ingredient used and melts very well. Another non-dairy cheese alternative is made by the Daiyafoods Co., www.daiyafoods.com. They make a delicious cheese alternative that is dairy-free, soy-free, and is used just like dairy cheese with the same results but without the harmful cholesterol, trans-fat or animal fat.

- **Non-dairy Mayo:** Followyourheart also makes *Vegenaise*, an awesome alternative to egg based mayo. No cholesterol, too.
- **Rice/Soy/Coconut Ice Creams:** Very good in flavor and texture. You will not miss dairy ice cream. Raw, non-dairy, non-soy are awesome. (See recipes.) You will have to taste the raw ones, then you will know what I mean when I say, unbelievably good.
- **Non-Dairy Sour and Cream Cheese:** Non-animal source substitutes, use as you would with dairy based ingredients.
- **Vegan Margarine:** A non-dairy alternative to butter and conventional margarine. Conventional margarine contains trans-fats, so avoid it. The non-dairy versions do not contain trans-fats. *EarthBalance* is a good company for non-dairy, non-trans fat margarines. Soy-free is also available.
- **Olive Oil Butter:** A good, healthy alternative to dairy butter and conventional margarine is olive oil. Simply put ½ cup of olive oil mixed with ½ teaspoon Himalayan salt, place in container and put in freezer. This makes a good tasting, high nutrient-based butter alternative. Use as you would traditional butter. Add a touch of crushed garlic for garlic olive oil butter.

<u>Meat Substitutes:</u>

There are several companies that make meat-like substitutes that are good protein sources and fortified with vitamins and minerals:

- **Tofu:** A good source of protein, calcium and other minerals. Texture varieties are soft, medium, firm and extra firm. Use just like you would animal flesh, in cooking recipes, sandwiches and salads. Seasoning is the key to tofu, as it will take on the flavor of the seasoning you are using. Plain is just that, plain, and a bad way to introduce someone to tofu.
- **Seitan:** (wheat gluten) The high protein part of wheat, seitan is low fat, cholesterol free with a meat-like texture. Use it in stir-fry, sandwiches, salads, soups or by itself. *Whitewave* brand is very good. Also the *Field Roast Grain Meat Co.* makes outstanding veggie meats and sausages. Meat eaters will love them!

- **Mushrooms:** Our fungi friends make a great substitute for animal flesh in recipes. Stir Fry, casseroles, salads and even sandwiches.
- **Soy-based Lunch Meats, Sausages, and Chilies:** Soy is used to make the majority of meat substitute items. You will find them in the chilled and frozen sections of the store.
- **Tempeh:** Is a nutritious fermented cake of beans and/or grains that has been eaten for centuries. *Turtle Island Foods* makes a wonderful 5-grain tempeh (soy beans, rice, millet, sunflower and sesame seeds) and other non-meat items.

A word on soy:

Research indicates that soy is good for our health. However, there is still some debate if soy is not so good for us. I use soy in my diet without worry, but remember that soy is just one of the beans and no one food should dominate your diet. Therefore, be sure to eat a variety of different plant-based foods and do not just polarize to using soy-based items because they make good meat substitutes.

Nature did not make any one food item more important than the others, so eat a variety. Nature made all the colors of the rainbow in plants, so eat all the colors and you will find your pot of gold of health.

Egg Replacing:

Approximately 70% of the calories in eggs are from animal fat. They are also loaded with cholesterol. So cutting back or even omitting eggs from your diet is probably better for your health. If a recipe has one or two eggs in it, you can usually just skip the eggs and add a couple tablespoons of water to the recipe. Other replacement ideas:

- *Ener-G Egg Replacer* (Boxed item found at natural food stores.)
- 1 heaping tablespoon of cornstarch with 2 tablespoons of water.
- 1 Banana for cakes, ½ for muffins or cookies.

Other recipe necessities:

- **Cacao:** A relatively unknown health gem to the US population, Cacao is full of antioxidants. Found in natural health food stores, it comes in whole bean, nibs, powder, and cacao butter. Once you start eating cacao, you will discover "Nature's true chocolate."
- **Miso:** Used for thousands of years, miso is a fermented food from rice, barley or soybeans. High in protein, vitamins and minerals, miso will add great flavor and nutrients to your recipes. Use only organic, unpasteurized and GMO-free miso. Comes in brown, yellow and red.
- **Nama Shoyu:** Raw, unpasteurized soy sauce, full of enzymes and lactobacillus (good for you). Under the *Ohsawa* brand, this is the real soy sauce and will forever change your taste buds for the better. You will never want cheap, rotgut soy sauce packets again. Wheat-free is available as well, under the *San-J* Platinum label.
- **Bragg's Liquid Aminos:** A certified non-GMO liquid protein concentrate, derived from healthy soybeans. Contains the essential and non-essential Amino Acids in naturally occurring amounts. Use in dressings, sauces, and stir-fry.
- **Lecithin (non-GMO):** Powder/granule form, found at natural food stores. Use in recipes to help bind ingredients. Anti-cholesterol properties and high in B vitamins.
- **Sea Vegetables:** Sea vegetables are full of nutrients, like iodine and other trace minerals. Added to your diet, brings health and taste.
  - **Dulce and Nori:** Can be eaten as a snack. Nori is used as a wrap in sushi making.
  - **Arame and Hijiki:** Simply soak, rinse and toss into a salad mix.
  - **Irish Moss:** Used to thicken and bind desserts. Rinse and soak overnight before using.
  - **Wakame:** Green and slippery with mild flavor. Use in soups and salads. New studies show Wakame is a fat burner...☺

- **Sweeteners:** We all love sweets. However, conventionally refined sugars (white, brown sugars, high-fructose corn syrup) are not good for you. **Artificial sweeteners should never be used.** Sugar-free "diet" foods, diet sodas and diet packet "sweeteners" are toxic to your system, and cause inflammation and bloating within your body. They do not help you burn fat, lose weight or increase your health. Don't let catchy marketing fool you into eating poisons. Chemical are NOT food.

Better sweeteners to use:

- **Raw Organic Agave Nectar:** From the cactus like plant, agave is a great natural sweetener. Use in nearly everything where sweetener is needed.
- **Dates:** Raw organic dates are wonderfully balanced with nutrients and flavor, but not overpowering so they work well in smoothies and recipes where a little sweetness is needed.
- **Maple Syrup:** Good sweetener that is not overpowering.
- **Sucanat:** Non-refined cane sugar. Highest nutrient content. Far better than refined sugars.

You can generally substitute 1 to 1 ratio of one sweetener for another. Example: ¼ cup agave for ¼ cup dates for ¼ cup maple syrup.

There is a "diet" drink with no toxic artificial sweetener. Made by *Steaz*, it is low-cal, low-sugar and no toxins. For those of you hooked on "diet" sodas, try *Steaz* brand (www.steaz.com).

Other pantry/freezer items to keep on hand:

Vegetable Stock: Use in place of animal based stocks. Use in soups, sauces and gravies. I like the organic pre-made vegetable stock by Pacificfoods. Usually come in 32 ounce carton.

Pre-Made Frozen Meals and Boxed items: The 16/21 Diet Solution provides you with many quick, easy-to-do recipes that are better than anything pre-made. However, time can be short or you may not feel like preparing food when you get home. If you want to use a pre-made frozen or a quick out of a box meal, there are better companies to use. Health conscious companies use more organic whole food ingredients in their products than the conventional, heavily processed methods. The organic whole food ingredients, make for a healthier, better tasting quick meal.

A few of the good companies are: *Casbah*, *Near East* and *Eden Foods* make very good canned and easy to prepare boxed items. *Amy's and StarLite* make frozen non-dairy items that are awesome. *Rising Moon* brand makes wonderful vegan ravioli's found in the frozen section of most health food stores.

For a list of recommended health food companies and their contact information; see Appendix B: Company List at the back of this book.

NOTE: There are some meat and dairy alternative food products on the market that are highly processed that I consider junk food. When using pre-made food products, the idea is to substitute healthier plant based food products in place of animal based products. However, I do not recommend you eat a diet that is filled with pre-made, processed products of and kind, plant or animal based. A healthy, successful diet must contain a daily intake of fresh unprocessed nutrient-rich foods.

The Real World Big Picture:

- Eating raw fruits, vegetables, nuts, and seeds provides you with great tasting, highly nutritious foods.
- Using whole grains instead of refined products will add health benefits and more satisfying meals, as they are not full of "empty" calories.
- The 16/21 Diet Solution provides you with complete meals—no skimping, no starving, and no loss of taste.
- The myth that "healthy food tastes bland" will fall like a ton of bricks.
- Preparing real food meals is quicker and easier than you thought.
- Leftovers are not just left-overs in The 16/21 Diet Solution. They are awesome meals to be eaten at work, school, or at 2 am after a night on the town.
- Studies show eating foods designed for you that are plant-based can provide you with numerous health benefits:

    1. Lower blood pressure
    2. Decrease risk of heart disease and cancers
    3. Permanent weight loss
    4. Reversal or prevention of diabetes
    5. Increased and more balanced energy levels
    6. Reduce and eliminate chronic inflammation

The 16/21 Diet Solution was designed for real people, just like you. Therefore, you can do it and you will love it!

CHAPTER 8

The Recipes

These recipes are great tasting, rich in nutrients and kid tested. Yes, my children have been the "testers" for my awesome, pretty good, interesting and pathetically bad recipes, since they were born. These recipes have all passed the test of even the pickiest of eaters. Kid tested, Doctor approved...Enjoy… ☺

After trying these recipes, and once you feel comfortable in using real foods predominately in your diet, get creative with them. Check my website for other recipes that are available for download.
Go to www.DocEmerson.com.

> **Note:** Caloric value, fat, carb, and protein values are listed on everything you purchase. I don't use them when referring to real food. A Twinkie will even list these values. What for? It's a Twinkie.
>
> It is my hope that you adopt the understanding that eating real food will lessen your need to keep the diet stats. These real food recipes are nutritious. Let your body experience nature's work.

Tips, Ideas and Guidelines:

Remember, the key to healthy eating is to eat real food as often as you can. Though it may sound difficult in the beginning, you can transform your kitchen into an easy working space with minimal effort and minimal expense. Using airtight containers like Pyrex glassware with sealable lids will make your kitchen, fridge, and your preparation organized and seamless. Think of your kitchen and fridge as an efficient, high-end restaurant. Airtight containers will make organization a snap.

Simply pull something from the fridge and presto, a quick and easy recipe is ready in minutes. You will find your fridge is quite large when there is less processed, packaged, bottled, and boxed products taking up the space and more real foods are stored inside.

- Turn the most time-consuming duties of recipe making into a 1-2 time per week event. Like washing produce, cooking rice, etc.
- Brown rice will store easily in an airtight container and will keep in the fridge to use all week. Make 10-12 cups at a time, once or twice a week in your rice cooker, as this will make meal prep quick and easy.
- Most nuts and seeds should be soaked overnight. After soaking, drain the soaking water and pour down the drain. Rinse the nuts or seeds in fresh water. Simply pat them dry with a paper towel and place in airtight container in the fridge, and they are ready to go for your next quick recipe.
- The dressings, hummus/spreads and sauces will keep several days in the fridge in an airtight container to use daily.
- Do your shredding of vegetables like carrots, zucchini, and beets during your meal prep. I recommend not shredding days beforehand, as you want fresh nutrients for your meal.
- Most all of my recipes are designed to make plenty of food for leftovers. Having awesome food ready to go for tomorrow's breakfast or lunch is a great time-saver. If you have a ton of kids like I do, then double the recipes so you have plenty of food for the next meal. Don't plan on storing leftovers for a week. Eat them the next day for best results, flavor and nutrient retention.
- Eating **real food** is our goal, not following what industry "standards" tells us what breakfast, lunch and dinners consist of. Therefore, I believe you can eat any of these recipes for any meal and truly enjoy them. Black Pepper Grits is one of my family's favorite dinners and enchiladas are great in the mornings.

- Smoothies can be made and eaten at breakfast and then taken to work or school in a "to go" container. Drop a couple ice cubes in as you leave the house and simply shake or stir again for a mid-morning snack.
- Once again, I am not advocating over-eating, but when you look at many product packages, most list ¼ to ½ cup as a serving size. No one eats a ¼ cup of anything and feels full and satisfied. My serving sizes are for real people.
- Eating real foods will allow you to eat well, enjoy flavors and not worry about portion size. Your body was designed for real foods and when you eat for your nutrient requirements, you will have a wonderful good feeling of fulfillment. Not the standard, "Oh my gosh, why did I eat so much, I can't breathe now."
- The number of servings listed per recipe is estimated. Through application, you will gauge you and your family's needs. For instance, during the high school football season, my recipes were always doubled and sometimes tripled so that there were plenty of wraps, enchiladas, salads and smoothies on hand.
- By using **real food**, your meals will never be boring. Be creative and by using **raw living foods**, there are no wrong combinations. You will become a master of food prep and creations in no time.
- The learning curve is always present starting something new, so try a recipe several times before you ban it...☺
- Another beautiful aspect of eating and cooking cleaner is clean-up. Your pans will not have the usual baked-on residue from cooking. Animal tissues are very "sticky" to your arteries as well as your pans. You will find my recipes are easy to make and just as easy to clean up afterwards. By washing fresh organic produce before use, food-borne illnesses in your kitchen will be pretty remote. Nearly every food-borne illness is linked to animal products.
  Remember, animal foods are comprised of the flesh and body

fluids of the animal. This means you are eating the fluids, bacterium, viruses, parasites and anything else that animal may have lurking inside of it. I advise you to make your kitchen area an "animal tissue-free zone" for cleaner living. If you want to eat the animal meal, you can always go to a restaurant and let them deal with the messy, sticky clean-up.☺

Measurement Conversion Chart

Cup	Fluid Oz	Tablespoon	Teaspoon	Milliliters	F° - C°
1/8 c	1 oz	2 tbsp	6 tsp	30 ml	225-110
1/4 c	2 oz	4 tbsp	12 tsp	59 ml	250-130
1/3 c	3 oz	6 tbsp	16 tsp	79 ml	275-140
1/2 c	4 oz	8 tbsp	24 tsp	118 ml	300-150
2/3 c	5 oz	11 tbsp	32 tsp	158 ml	325-170
3/4 c	6 oz	12 tbsp	36 tsp	177 ml	350-180
1 c	8 oz	16 tbsp	48 tsp	237 ml	375-190
2 c	16 oz	32 tbsp	96 tsp	473 ml	400-200
Cup	**Fluid Oz**	**Pint**	**Quart**	**Liters**	
2 c	16 oz	1 pt	1/2 qt	.473 L	425-220
4 c	32 oz	2 pts	1 qt	.95 L	450-230
16 c	1 gal	8 pts	4 qts	3.79 L	475-240

Power House Smoothies

Smoothies are a great way to get a lot of nutrients and a good energy source. These recipes **do not need** additional protein powders, weight loss mixes, eye of newt, bone chunks, pixie dust or anything else other than natural ingredients listed. Enjoy them as a snack or even a quick meal. Way better than a bag of chemical-induced chips.

Green Power

4 Organic Bananas

1 cup Organic Raw Spinach

2 cups Filtered Water

1 Tablespoon Organic Raw Agave Nectar

Blend together on high for about 1 minute. Serves 2-3.

Berry Green Power

4 Organic Bananas

1 cup Organic Raw Spinach

2 cups Filtered Water

1 cup Organic Blueberries

½ cup Organic Blackberries

1 Tablespoon Organic Raw Agave Nectar

Blend together on high for about 1 minute. Serves 2-3.

Banango

2 cups Coconut Water (one young/immature coconut)

2 Organic Bananas

1 Whole Mango (peeled, seed removed)

1 Tablespoon Organic Raw Agave Nectar

Blend together on high for about 1 minute. Serves 2-3.

Berry-Choco Smoothie

2 cups Filtered Water

2 cups Organic Strawberries or Raspberries

2 Organic Bananas

2 Tablespoons Organic Raw Cacao Powder

1 Tablespoon Vanilla Extract

2 Tablespoons Organic Raw Agave Nectar

½ cup Organic Raw Almonds, soaked overnight

Handful of Ice Cubes

Blend together on high for about 1 minute. Serves 2-3.

Bananacado Smoothie

4-5 Organic Bananas

2 cups Filtered Water

1 Avocado, peeled and pitted

1 Tablespoon Organic Raw Agave Nectar

Blend well to desired consistency. Serves 2-3.

Berry Nut Smoothie

2 cups Filtered Water

1 cup Organic Cashews, soaked overnight

1 teaspoon Vanilla Extract

2 cups Organic Strawberries or Raspberries

1 Tablespoon Organic Raw Agave Nectar

Blend together on high for about 1 minute. Serves 2-3.

Orange Juice Sunrise

1 cup Ice Cubes

3 cups fresh Squeezed Organic Orange Juice

1 ripe Organic Banana

Blend until smooth. Serves 3.

Macadamia Nut Berry Smoothie

2 cups Filtered Water

1/2 cup Macadamia Nuts, not soaked

1 teaspoon Vanilla Extract

2 cups Organic Strawberries or Raspberries

1 Tablespoon Organic Raw Agave Nectar

Blend together on high for about 1 minute. Serves 2-3.

Coconut Almond Smoothie

2 cups Coconut Water (one young/immature coconut)

Coconut meat from the Coconut

3 heaping Tablespoons Organic Raw Almond Butter

4-5 Organic Dates pitted

1 Tablespoon Organic Raw Agave Nectar

½ teaspoon Vanilla

Pinch Himalayan Pink Salt

5-6 large Ice Cubes

Place all ingredients in blender and blend until smooth.

The Power of Juicing

Fresh, raw organic juices are very nutritious and good for you. I have heard all sorts of odd ideas as to why fresh, raw juice is not good. "There is too much sugars in raw juice; too concentrated; they make you fat," but none of these odd claims have merit. So, compared to a soda, diet soda or a "juice" drink with 10% "real" juice, the fresh, raw organic juice is good for you, period! Wash all ingredients before use.

Pineapple Juice (huge anti-inflammatory)

1 whole Organic Pineapple washed, with top off, cut into strips

Juice the entire pineapple, skin and all. One ripe pineapple should yield 24-26 ounces of juice.

If you are experiencing pains or illness. Drink 10-12 oz upon arising, and 10-12 oounces 2 hours before bed.

Digestion Cooler

4-5 Organic Carrots

1 3-inch wedge of Organic Green Cabbage

½ Organic Apple

Juice everything together. Yields 10-12 ounces.

Carrot/Apple Juice

4-5 large Organic Carrots

½ Organic Apple

Juice everything together. Yields 10-12 ounces.

Blood Purifier Carrot/Beet Juice

4-5 Large Organic Carrots

½ Organic Beet

1 clove Garlic

Hand-full of Raw Parsley (optional)

Juice everything together. Yields 10-12 ounces.

There are many good juicing recipes available. I believe in the power of juices and recommend you try many recipes and make some of your own. When using greens, use ¼ greens to ¾ carrots. Carrots make a solid base for any juice. Get creative.

Healthy Cooking Notes & Recipe Creating Tips:

It is important to eliminate **conventionally refined oils** in your diet as often as possible, as they are treated with chemicals and probably genetically engineered. Therefore, I recommend that you use **organic unrefined oils** exclusively. I usually do not use high heat temps for cooking, so the low, medium and medium-high temps are generally OK for unrefined oils. I recommend you use a variety of different oils, experiment and be creative with them. Many of the wonderful **organic unrefined oils** include:

- Avocado
- Almond
- Apricot
- Coconut
- Hazelnut
- Olive
- Palm
- Safflower
- Sunflower
- Sesame
- Toasted Sesame
- Walnut

Do Not Heat: Borage, Evening Primrose, Flax or Hemp Oils. These oils are too delicate for heat. Use as a raw oil application only.

Genetically Modified Organism (GMO) or Genetically Engineered (GE):

I must repeat: Soy, corn, canola and cotton are the four most common genetically manipulated crops and are commonly used as cooking oils. The United States does not require disclosure labels on GE or GMO foods, as of yet. Currently there is **no federal regulation, except for USDA organic standards, which prohibit genetically engineered ingredients. That is why I am a stickler for organic.** They may cost a little more at the checkout line, but eating toxins is too high of a price topay with your health.

Organic is Best,
Non-Organic is ok when you have to,
GMO's should be avoided.

Dressings

Traditionally known as "salad" dressings, these versatile dressings can help dress veggies, pastas, rices, sandwiches, pitas and even burritos. Be as creative as you wish with different organic oils. Remember, nutrients is the key to health, so enjoy. Most conventional made dressings like ranch or thousand island have a lot of fat and chemical fillers for shelf life; you do not need that in your body. Fresh is always best and these are easy to make!

Anti-Inflammatory Dressing

½ cup Organic Unrefined Olive Oil

¼ cup Balsamic Vinegar

¼ cup Nama Shoyu

1 clove crushed Organic Garlic

Whisk together. Pour over choice of food. Serves 5-6. Store left over in airtight container in fridge.

Raw Tomatahini Dressing

10 Organic Grape Tomatoes

¼ cup Organic Raw Tahini

¼ cup Nama Shoyu

Organic Lime Juice, a couple squeezes

Blend together. Pour over food. Serves 6.

Note for Recipe Ingredients;

* Nama Shoyu is soy sauce that is unpasteurized. It contains wheat.
* San-J Platinum Label Brand is wheat-free and reduced sodium.
* Bragg's Liquid Aminos is a certified Non-GMO liquid protein made from soybeans and contains essential amino acids.

I prefer Nama Shoyu, San-J Platinum Brand and/or Bragg's Liquid Aminos in my recipes due to their rich flavor and higher nutrient content. I do not add salt to the recipes that contain these sauces.

Basil Pine Nut / Almond Dressing

1 cup Pine Nuts, (not soaked)

1 cup Filtered Water

2 cups Fresh Organic Basil

1 Tablespoon Nama Shoyu

¼ cup Organic Almonds, soaked overnight

Blend all ingredients together until creamy. Serves 5-6.

Peanut-Curry Dressing

1 cup Organic Roasted Peanuts

1 clove Organic Garlic

1 small piece Organic Ginger

1 teaspoon Curry Powder

1 ½ cups Water

1 Tablespoon Nama Shoyu

1 Tablespoon Toasted Sesame Oil

Blend together until smooth. Makes about two cups, serves 6.

Salads

Nearly anything fresh and plant-based can be a salad in my kitchen. Side salads in restaurants, are many times an after thought, and to kids they are as bad as cell phones that can't text. But when you make them versatile, they become very enjoyable and even a complete meal. So, be creative and use anything you that is from the **16/21** list to make a salad.

All-Star Salad

Large mixing bowl of Organic Mixed Greens

1 Organic Cucumber, chopped

1 Avocado, peeled, pitted and diced

10 Organic Cherry Tomatoes (green, red or yellow)

1 cup Organic Raw Okra, chopped

Toss together. Serve. Enjoy! Serves 1-2.

Veggie Salad (lettuce free salad)

2 Organic Carrots, shredded

1 Organic Zucchini, shredded

1 Organic Beet, shredded

½ Head of Organic Cabbage, shredded

1 cup Organic Corn

Toss with dressing of choice. Serves 2-3.

Avo-Cucumber Salad

5-6 Avocados, peeled, pitted, and cubed

4 Organic Cucumbers, sliced

1 basket of Organic Cherry Tomatoes

3 Green Onions, chopped

2 sprigs Fresh Rosemary Leaves, stems removed

2 Tablespoons Organic Raw Tahini

¼ cup Organic Unrefined Olive Oil

2 Tablespoons Bragg's Liquid Aminos

1 clove crushed Organic Garlic

1 Tablespoon Fresh Crushed Black Pepper

Combine olive oil, Bragg's, raw tahini, pepper, and garlic in a cup and mix well. Place veggies in large bowl, and liquid mix and toss. Serves 4.

Salad ideas and variations: Sauté seitanover medium heat in avocado oil with crushed garlic for 4-5 minutes, then toss in salad.

Kale / Wakame Salad

1 bunch of Organic Kale

1 package Dried Wakame

1 cup Shiitake Mushrooms, sliced

½ cup Nama Shoyu

3 Tablespoons Bragg's Liquid Aminos

¼ teaspoon Crushed Organic Garlic

2 Tablespoons Bragg's Apple Cider Vinegar

¼ teaspoon Minced Organic Ginger

1 Avocado, peeled, pitted and cubed

¼ cup Pine Nuts, (not soaked)

¼ cup Filtered Water

Cut Kale leaves from stem and slice leaves into long thin strips. Cut dried wakame into long thin strips as well. (Scissors work great.) In a small bowl soak dried wakame in cool fresh water for 10 minutes, drain, rinse well again. Wakame may have a slight salty sea taste.

In medium bowl, mix Nama Shoyu, Bragg's Aminos, apple cider vinegar, ginger, garlic and water together. Add mushrooms and marinate 10 minutes. Add kale and wakame to mixture and toss well. Garnish with avocado cubes, pine nuts, Himalayan salt and pepper. Serves 4.

Hummus and Spreads

Hummus and spreads are a great way to add nutrients and great taste to your diet. Use them as dips, dressings or condiments. Substitute for egg mayonnaise, butter, milk, and sour cream based items. These recipes are awesome on whole grain toast or even by themselves. Once again, get creative and enjoy.

Black-Eyed Pea Hummus

2 (15 oz) cans Organic Black-Eyed Peas, drained

2 cloves Raw Organic Garlic

Pinch Himalayan Pink Salt

¼ cup Organic Unrefined Olive Oil

Blend together to desired consistency in blender or food processor. Serves 3-4.

Baby Lima Bean / Sun Dried Hummus

2 (15 oz) cans Organic Baby Lima Beans, drained

1 clove Raw Organic Garlic

¼ cup Sun Dried Tomatoes, chopped (pre-soak in hot water for 15 mins)

¼ cup Organic Green Onion, chopped

Pinch Himalayan Pink Salt

¼ cup Organic Unrefined Walnut Oil

Blend together to desired consistency in blender or food processor. Serves 4-5.

Rosemary Artichoke Hummus

1 (14 oz) can Artichoke Hearts packed in water, drained

1 clove Organic Garlic

Pinch Himalayan Pink Salt

1 can Pitted Jumbo Black Olives, drained

1 sprig of fresh Organic Rosemary Leaves, stem removed

¼ cup Organic Unrefined Walnut Oil

Blend together to desired consistency in blender or food processor. Serves 3-4.

Sunflower Power

2 cups Raw Organic Sunflower Seeds, soaked overnight

1 cup Sun Dried Tomatoes, chopped, (pre-soak in hot water for 15 mins)

½ cup Fresh Organic Cilantro

2 raw Organic Garlic Cloves

½ Jalapeno Pepper, diced (seeds removed)

1 Tablespoon Organic Brown Miso, unpasteurized

¼ teaspoon Himalayan Pink Salt

1 teaspoon Fresh Crushed Black Pepper

2 teaspoons Organic Cayenne Powder

1 Avocado, peeled and pitted

Blend together to desired consistency. Serves 5-6.

Avo-Delight

2 ripe Avocados, peeled and pitted

½ clove Organic Garlic

¼ teaspoon Himalayan Pink Salt

1 teaspoon Fresh Crushed Black Pepper

Mash together in bowl to blend. Serves 2-3

A quick option is to chop 2 Roma tomatoes and add ¼ teaspoon Turmeric added to avocado, then mix well.

Cream Cheese (healthy with no guilt)

This cream cheese is rich in minerals, vitamins and essential fatty acids.

2 cups Organic Raw Cashews, soaked overnight

3 Tablespoons Extra Virgin Olive Oil

¼ cup Organic Lemon juice, fresh squeezed

¾ teaspoon Himalayan Pink Salt

1 cup Filtered Water

Combine all ingredients in food processor and blend until creamy. Use water to thin to your desired consistency. Add a tablespoon of water at a time.

For flavored cream cheese, add chopped onions and/or couple garlic cloves while blending.

Soups

These soups are easy to make and very nutritious. They are quick, **raw** and don't need to be cooked, simply serve after blending. If you prefer a little warmth to your soup, warm in saucepan over medium heat for 2-3 minutes.

Raw Avochini Soup

3 Organic Zucchinis, chopped

2 Avocados, peeled, pitted and diced

1 cup Filtered Water

3 Tablespoons Organic Unrefined Olive Oil

¼ cup Organic Fresh Oregano; use dried if fresh is not available

3 cloves Organic Garlic

½ teaspoon Himalayan Pink Salt

1 teaspoon Fresh Crushed Black Pepper

Fresh Organic Chives, chopped

1 Organic Carrot, shredded

Blend until smooth in food processor or blender. Garnish with shredded carrots and chopped chives.

Also can be used as a sauce over vegetables or whole grain pasta.

Raw Caliente Soup

6 Avocados, peeled and pitted

4-5 Organic Roma Tomatoes, chopped

1 cup Organic Celery, chopped

½ Jalapeno Pepper, chopped (seeds removed)

4-5 Organic Green Onions

½ cup Fresh Organic Cilantro

4 Tablespoons Fresh Lemon Juice

½ Habenero Pepper, chopped (seeds removed)

½ teaspoon Himalayan Pink Salt

Blend until smooth in food processor or blender. Garnish with pieces of cilantro. Serves 4.

Shiitake Mushroom Soup

3 Tablespoons Brown Rice Miso, unpasteurized

1 cup Organic Unrefined Olive Oil

2 cloves Organic Garlic

3 cups Filtered Water

3 Organic Green Onions, chopped

3 cups Shiitake Mushrooms, sliced

½ cup Nama Shoyu

In mixing bowl, marinade mushrooms with ½ cup Nama Shoyu for approximately 20 minutes. Blend together remaining ingredients in blender until smooth. Add mushrooms to blended mixture. Serves 4.

Variation: Add cooked soba noodles to Shiitake soup and serve slightly warm or cold.

Soup for What Ails Ya'

7 cups of Filtered water

2 cups Organic Vegetable Stock (*Pacific Foods* brand)

3 Tablespoons Organic Brown Rice Miso, unpasteurized

1 cup Nama Shoyu

¼ cup Bragg's Liquid Aminos

2 cups Fresh Shiitake Mushrooms, sliced

6-7 slices of fresh Organic Ginger or fresh grated

10-12 cloves Organic Garlic, peeled and crushed

5-6 leaves of fresh Organic Basil, chopped

1 handful of fresh Organic Parsley, chopped

4 Organic Green Onions, chopped

1 teaspoon Crushed Black Pepper

1-2 (8 oz) packages of Organic Soba Noodles (*Organic Planet* brand)

Place all ingredients, except noodles in a large pot. Mix well and cook on medium heat for 5 minutes. Add noodles and continue to simmer for another 8-10 minutes to cook noodles. Serves 4.

Sauces

A great tasting recipe is dependent upon the sauce. Would a meat dish taste edible without the base or sauce? Plain baked chicken breast is terrible and everyone who has tried that diet knows this. My sauces are packed with nutrient-rich ingredients and taste great. Use as dressing for salads, dip for veggies, a spread for whole grain breads, or toss with whole grain pastas or brown rice. Sauces, similar to dressings, are versatile and another great way to add a lot of nutrients to your meal. Using all fresh, organic ingredients, you will see the difference in health and taste.

Pesto Guarendo (Healing Pesto)

3 cups Raw Organic Sunflower Seeds, soaked overnight

¼ cup Pine Nuts

1 cup Fresh Organic Basil

¼ cup Olive Oil or Walnut Oil

½ teaspoon Himalayan Pink Salt

1 teaspoon Curshed Black Pepper

1 Organic Lemon, squeezed by hand

Blend until smooth in food processor or blender to desired consistency. Serves 4. Use as a sauce, dip or spread on whole grain breads.

Nut Sauce

¼ cup Pine Nuts

½ cup Organic Cashews, soaked overnight

½ cup Macadamia Nuts, (mac nuts do not need soaking)

¼ cup Organic Unrefined Walnut Oil

2 cloves Organic Garlic

2 Tablespoons Nama Shoyu

1 cup Filtered Water, for thinning

Blend until smooth in food processor or blender. Thin with water for desired consistency. Serves 4.

Peanut Sauce

2 Tablespoons Organic Raw Tahini

2 Tablespoons Organic Brown Rice Miso, unpasteurized

2 Tablespoons Nama Shoyu

1 cup Raw Organic Peanuts, or use roasted if you prefer

1 Tablespoon Organic Raw Agave Nectar

4 Tablespoons Fresh Squeezed Orange Juice

1 Tablespoon Red Chili Flakes

1 cup Filtered Water

Blend until smooth in food processor or blender. Thin with water to desired consistency. Serves 4.

Roma-Basil Sauce

1 cup Fresh Organic Basil

4-5 quartered Fresh Organic Roma Tomatoes

½ cup Organic Unrefined Olive Oil

3 cloves Organic Garlic

1 Tablespoon Fresh Black Pepper

½ teaspoon Himalayan Pink Salt

½ cup Filtered Water

Blend until smooth in food processor or blender. Thin with water for desired consistency.

Entrees

As a parent who raised a bunch of kids, I am a firm believer in getting the MOST out of a meal. Since kids love quick meals, too, I discovered it is possible to WRAP anything that is highly nutritious into a whole grain tortilla and literally make a complete meal out of it. It is fast food without the junk.

Wrap-O-Meal

½ of a (1 lb.) box of pre-washed Organic Mixed Greens (*Earthbound Farms*, found at Costco, Whole Foods, and most major markets)

4 cups Organic Brown Rice or Quinoa, cooked

1 (15 oz) can Organic Corn, drained

1 (15 oz) can Organic Baby Lima Beans, drained

4 Organic Roma Tomatoes, chopped

3 Organic Green Onions, chopped

1 cup Raw Organic Broccoli, chopped into small pieces

1 cup Raw Organic Cauliflower, chopped into small pieces

1 cup Shiitake Mushrooms, sliced (sliced portabella are awesome, too)

6 extra-large Organic Tortillas (Whole Foods Market sells individual XL tortillas at their burrito bar for about a .75 cents each.)

2 cloves Garlic, crushed

3 Tablespoons Sunflower Oil

3 Tablespoons Bragg's Liquid Aminos

2 Avocados, peeld, pitted, mashed up in bowl with Himalayan Pink Salt & Crushed Black Pepper

6 sheets of Foil Wrap

Preheat Oven to 375° F.

In a large pan, heat sunflower oil on medium heat; mix crushed garlic and 3 Tablespoons of Bragg's Liquid Aminos into oil. Add mushrooms and onions and sauté for 3-4 minutes. Add Brown rice, corn, lima beans, broccoli, cauliflower and tomatoes to pan, mix together well, and cook to heat all ingredients for another 4-5 minutes.

Lay tortilla out flat. Add large handful of mixed greens and kitchen spoon size amount of ingredients from pan onto tortilla. Simply roll tortilla ¾ of the way, tuck each end toward center of roll and continue to roll complete. Wrap in foil and place on oven rack for 5-10 minutes to warm wraps. Dress with avocado mix after heating in oven. Enjoy!

This wrap has everything you need for a complete meal. Low in fat, and high in nutrients, protein, complex carbs and greens. This is a satisfying meal.

Alternate ideas: Substitute legume choices with Organic Black-Eyed Peas, Pintos, Black Beans, Adzuki

Add Sunflower Sprouts.

Add 1 package of Seitan to the cooking mixture.

Add salsa.

You can also double the recipe and make 12 wraps so you have breakfast or lunches made for tomorrow that are ready to go!

Jack Talk Thai (Raw Version)

Inspired by one of my favorite Thai Restaurants in Tampa, Florida, and sentimentally named after a line used by the movie character Gaylord Focker.

1 cup Organic Cauliflower, chopped

1 cup Organic Broccoli, chopped

1 Organic Green Bell Pepper, diced

1 Organic Red Bell Pepper, diced

1 cup Shiitake Mushrooms, sliced

1 Bunch Organic Green Onions, chopped

Place all ingredients in bowl. Set aside and make raw sauce.

The Raw Sauce

1 cup Coconut Meat from Immature Coconut

1 cup Coconut Water from Immature Coconut

2 Tablespoons Organic Raw Tahini

2 Tablespoons Nama Shoyu

3 Organic Garlic Cloves

1 small Organic Ginger, diced

1 teaspoon Chili Flakes

½ teaspoon Turmeric Powder

1 teaspoon Organic Raw Agave Nectar

Blend until Smooth. Pour over the bowl of veggies and toss. Serves 6.

(See pages 136-138 for mastering the extraction of coconut water and meat.)

Jack Talk Thai (Cooked Version)

1 cup Organic Broccoli, chopped

1 cup Organic Cauliflower, chopped

1 Organic Red Bell Pepper, diced

1 cup Shiitake Mushrooms, sliced

1 package Seitan, chopped (*Whitewave* or *Sweet Earth* brand)

½ cup Organic Unrefined Walnut Oil

¼ cup Bragg's Liquid Aminos

In large sauce pan, heat with walnut oil and Bragg's Aminos on medium heat. When hot, sauté ingredients together until lightly cooked approx. 5-10 minutes.

The Cooked Sauce

1 cup Coconut Meat

1 cup Coconut Water

(1 can of Coconut Milk & 1 cup filtered water can be substituted for fresh Coconut Meat and Coconut Water in cooked version)

2 Tablespoons Nama Shoyu

2 Tablespoons Organic Raw Tahini

1 teaspoon Red Chili Flakes

½ teaspoon Turmeric Powder

1 teaspoon Organic Raw Agave Nectar

1 cup Organic Roasted Peanuts

3 Organic Garlic Cloves

3 cups of Organic Brown Rice or Quinoa, cooked

Add all ingredients except rice to blender and blend until smooth. Add blended mix to heating veggie pan and mix well. Continue to heat for two minutes over medium heat. Pour over brown rice or quinoa and serve.

Magic Mushrooms

1 lb. Fresh Mushrooms (button or baby portabellas), washed

½ cup Organic White Onions

1 cup Black Olives jumbo, pitted

2 Tablespoons Organic Unrefined Olive Oil or Avocado Oil

Handful of Fresh Organic Basil

1 Organic Red Bell Pepper, diced

Clean mushrooms; remove stems, set caps aside. In food processor, pulse to chop or use a blender to blend remaining ingredients until mixture is smooth. Place mixture onto mushroom caps. Drizzle a little oil and Himalayan Pink salt over mushrooms. Enjoy. Serves 3-4.

Variation: Use portabella mushrooms; cut stem and spoon out enough room in cap to place mixture inside.

Stuffed Red Peppers

3 cups Organic Sunflower Seeds, (soaked overnight)

1 ½ cups Sun Dried Tomatoes, soaked in warm water 15 minutes

½ cup Fresh Organic Cilantro

2 cloves Raw Organic Garlic

½ Jalapeno Pepper, seeds removed

1 Tablespoon Organic Brown Rice Miso, unpasteurized

4-5 Organic Red Bell Peppers (green or yellow), tops and seeds removed

2 teaspoon Cayenne Pepper

1 Avocado, peeled and pitted

½ teaspoon Himalayan Pink Salt

2 Tablespoons Crushed Black Pepper

Combine all ingredients except Red Bell Peppers into blender and blend until smooth. Stuff Red Peppers with mixture. Serves 4-5.

*Avocado Variation: Use 3-4 avocados and only 1 cup soaked sunflower seeds. The stuffed peppers can be wrapped in plastic wrap and stored in refrigerator for several days, and make great snacks as leftovers.

La Vita E'Buona (Life is Good - Raw)

No cooking required for this recipe. This is how food should taste.

The Fresh Raw Sauce:

8 Organic Roma Tomatoes

1 cup Sun-Dried Tomatoes, chopped (soaked in hot water 15 mins)

1 cup Fresh Organic Raw Basil

2 Organic Green Onions, chopped

¼ cup Organic Unrefined Olive Oil

1 Tablespoon Nama Shoyu

3 Organic Garlic Cloves

¼ cup Organic Raw Parsley

1 sprig Organic Rosemary Leaves, stem removed

½ teaspoon Himalayan Pink Salt

Add to Blender and blend well until sauce-like.

Fresh Raw "Pasta" (use veggies as the pasta):

Use a julienne to make the "pasta"

2 large Organic Zucchini, sliced into long thin strips

10 jumbo Pitted Olives, chopped

Cooked Pasta version:

Toss raw sauce with organic whole grain pasta, cooked al dente.
Serves 3-4.

Awesome Thai Enchiladas

4 cups Organic Brown Rice or Quinoa, cooked

2 cups Shiitake Mushrooms, sliced

(Marinate mushrooms in ¾ cup Nama Shoyu soy sauce in bowl while preparing rest of the meal)

1 package Seitan, chopped (*Whitewave* or *Sweet Earth* brand)

1 bunch Organic Green Onions, chopped

4 Organic Roma Tomatoes, diced into small pieces

4 packs of Organic Fat Free Flour Tortillas

2-3 cloves Organic Garlic, crushed

¼ cup Organic Unrefined Walnut Oil

Sauté seitan, tomatoes and onions in 1/8 cup walnut oil with pressed garlic for 3-4 minutes over medium heat. Then add marinated mushrooms with marinade sauce and brown rice, stir together and cook for 2-3 minutes. In fat-free flour tortillas, roll ingredients into enchiladas and place onto baking pan. Lightly coat rolled tortillas with remaining walnut oil and bake at 375° F for 10-12 minutes. Serves 10-12.

Miles' Famous Enchiladas

2 cups Organic Brown, Basmati, or Jade Green Rice, cooked

2 (15 oz) cans Enchilada Sauce (mild, medium, hot, your choice)

2 (14 oz) cans Artichoke Hearts (packed in water), drained and chopped

1 (28 oz) can Organic Diced Tomatoes, chopped more

1 can Pitted Jumbo Olives, chopped

1 package Vegan Mozzarella Cheese (*Follow Your Heart* brand), grated

2 packs Organic Fat-Free Flour Tortillas

Lightly oil casserole pans with sunflower oil and a little red sauce. Place a mixture of ingredients into tortilla and roll. Place each enchilada into pan and after pan is full, cover enchiladas with red sauce and remaining cheese. Bake at 375 for 15 minutes. Serve with salad, salsa, and avocado. Enjoy! Makes about 12-14 enchiladas. Serves 5-6.

A note about cooking whole grain pasta:

Whole grain pasta should not boil for very long. Bring water to boil on high, place the pasta into the boiling water, reduce heat to med/med-high and allow whole grain pasta to cook in hot water, but not boil the entire time. This will allow for better taste and more nutrients to be retained. Rinse with cold water immediately to stop the cooking process, drain and serve.

The Non-Believer's Alfredo

This is a great recipe for those of you who love creamy type sauces. This one has no cholesterol and is very tasty and provides wonderful comfort.

16 oz package Organic Whole Grain Penne Pasta

¼ cup Organic Soy-Free Margarine, non-hydrogenated (*Earth Balance*)

1 cup Vegan Mozzarella Cheese (*Follow Your Heart* brand), grated

¼ cup Organic Whole Wheat Pastry Flour

2 cups Organic Plain Soy Milk (or any "Nut Milk" that is unflavored, unsweetened)

½ cup Sun-Dried Tomatoes, soaked in hot water 15 minutes

2 cups Shiitake or Chanterelle Mushrooms, sliced

3 cloves Raw Organic Garlic, crushed

In a medium saucepan, over medium heat, heat ¼ soy margarine to liquefy state with the crushed garlic. Then add ½ cup of soy milk and ¼ cup flour, and stir while it thickens still on medium heat. You will add ½ cup of milk as the sauce thickens each time.

After all the "milk" is blended, add the chopped sun-dried tomatoes, vegan cheese and mushrooms. Stir until thickened again. Add salt and crushed pepper to taste. Boil the pasta at the same time as you are making the sauce. Serve sauce over pasta immediately and enjoy. Serves 4.

California Rolls

4 Nori Sheets

2 cups Alfalfa Sprouts

2 Avocados, pitted, peeled, and sliced

1 Organic Cucumber, cut lengthwise

2 cups Organic Brown Rice, cooked

1 cup warm Filtered Water

Dipping Sauce:

1 teaspoon Organic Brown Rice Miso, unpasteurized

1 teaspoon crushed Organic Garlic

4 Tablespoons Nama Shoyu

¼ teaspoon crushed Organic Ginger

¼ teaspoon Wasabi (optional)

It is helpful to have bamboo sushi mat, but not required. Lay Nori Sheet with shiny side down onto mat. Along edge of nori sheet closest to you, layer in ingredients. Roll mat; just before completing roll, dip your index finger into water and run it along the edge of the wrap. This will seal the wrap's seam. If no sushi mat is being used, you can roll the Nori sheet carefully by hand and seal the roll the same way. Cut into 5-6 pieces.

Weight Loss Wraps

6 Organic Collard Leaves

½ cup Organic Beets, grated

½ cup Organic Carrots, grated

2 Avocado, peeled and cut into slices

1 cup Sunflower Sprouts

1 Organic Cucumber, cut length wise into strips

Cut off thickest part of collard leaves stems. Lay Collard leaf out flat and layer vegetables onto leaves. Season with your favorite flavors, such as soy sauce, plum sauce, or salsa, Roll leaves into burritos style, tucking in the ends as you go. Slice in half. Yields 12 pieces. Serves 3-4.

Gabriela's Garlic Mashed Potatoes

12-16 medium sized Organic Red Potatoes

4 Organic Garlic Cloves

1 cup Organic Plain Soy Milk (unsweetened, unflavored)

½ cup Organic Unrefined Olive Oil

½ teaspoon Himalayan Pink Salt

1 teaspoon Crushed Black Pepper

In large stock pot, boil red potatoes with skins until tender. With large kitchen spoon, place cooked potatoes into blender and add garlic, olive oil, salt and pepper. Blend well. Add soy milk to thin to desired consistency. Serves 4-6.

If you have any leftovers from Gabriela's Mashed Potatoes, you can make either hash browns or potato pancakes. In a large skillet, heat suitable oil on medium-high heat. Spread potatoes out into 5-inch patties and brown for 3-4 minutes on each side or until your suited golden color. Serve with catsup, hot sauce, or a hint of the olive oil butter.

Bok Choy Actually Taste Great

3 Organic Baby Bok Choy, cut in quarters lengthwise

1 bunch Organic Kale or Swiss Chard, or both

1 package Organic Firm Tofu, cubed

2 cups Shiitake Mushrooms, sliced

1 Organic Yellow Pepper, chopped

1 cup Organic Broccoli, chopped

1 (32 oz) Organic Vegetable Broth (*Pacific Foods* brand)

4 Organic Green Onions, chopped

3 Cloves Organic Garlic

1 small piece Organic Raw Ginger

½ cup Bragg's Liquid Aminos

4 cups Organic Brown Rice or Quinoa, cooked

In large saucepan, heat 24 ounces of the vegetable broth and ¼ cup Bragg's Aminos over medium heat; add bok choy, kale and/or Swiss chard. Cover pan and allow to cook down until greens are soft and tender, approx 5-7 minutes. Do not overcook. Add onions, tofu, mushrooms, yellow pepper, and broccoli to pan and cook 3-4 minutes more. In blender, blend remaining vegetable broth, Bragg's Liquid Aminos, garlic, and ginger into sauce. Pour blender sauce into pan and mix well. Serve over Brown Rice or Quinoa.

Lasagna (Best Ever)

Imagine a lasagna with NO cholesterol and still tastes awesome!

1 (16 oz) box Organic Lasagna Noodles

2 (26 oz) jars Organic Pasta Sauce (dairy-free)

3 packs Vegan Mozzarella Cheese (*Daiya* Brand)

1 can Pitted Jumbo Olives, chopped

1 package Original Beef Substitute (*LifeLite* brand)

4 Organic Green Onions, chopped

6-7 Cloves of Organic Garlic

1 large and 1 medium-sized lasagna dishes

Boil Lasagna noodles until tender, drain in colander and rinse in cold water. Preheat oven to 375° F. Lightly coat entire bottom of lasagna pans with olive oil and pasta sauce mixture. Layer lasagna noodle side by side the length of pan. Cover noodle layer with pasta sauce, cover with meat then cheese. Continue with second layer of noodles; add pasta sauce, meat, cheese, onions and olives. Finish top layer with pasta sauce and cheese. Garnish top and sides of lasagna with cloves of garlic. Add fresh ground pepper and salt to taste. Cover assembled lasagna with foil and bake for 50 minutes at 375° F. Allow to cool and serve. This recipe makes one of the best leftover meals ever, too.

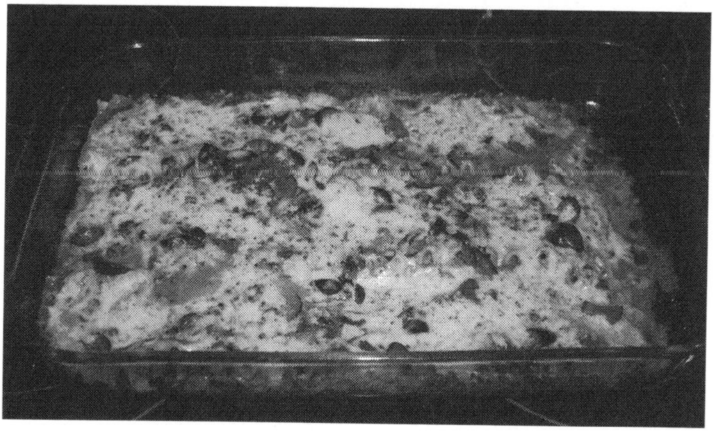

Best Lasagna Ever

Mushroom Stroganoff

2 cups Organic Vegetable Stock

12 oz Veggie Sour Cream (*Follow Your Heart* brand)

5-6 Organic Green Onions, chopped

½ pound Chanterelle Mushrooms, (shiitakes as alternative)

5 cloves Organic Garlic, chopped

4 Tablespoons Organic Whole Wheat Flour

¼ cup Organic Vegan Worcestershire Sauce (*The Wizard* brand)

2 cups Organic Broccoli, chopped

¼ cup Organic Unrefined Sunflower Oil

1 package Organic Whole Wheat Linguine

In large saucepan, heat oil and Worcestershire sauce (vegan) over medium heat, add crush garlic into warming oil. Heat for 2-3 minutes, then add green onions. Allow to cook 2-3 minutes more, then add mushrooms and broccoli. Add vegetable stock, flour, and vegan sour cream, stir well until blended. Simmer over low heat for 10-15 minutes. Allow sauce to thicken, stirring occasionally. Boil linguine for 7-8 minutes until al dente. Rinse in cold water and serve sauce over pasta. (Substitute any of your favorite mushrooms when chanterelles are not available.)

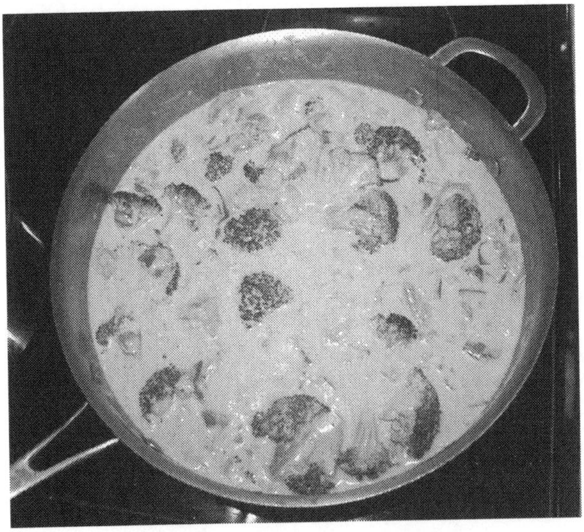

Mushroom Stroganoff ready to serve

Sandwiches

Hummus Burgers

2 cups cooked or 1 (15 oz) Organic Garbanzo Beans, mashed

1 Organic Carrot, finely chopped

¼ Organic Red Onion, chopped

¼ cup Organic Whole Wheat Flour

½ teaspoon each Himalayan Pink Salt & Crushed Black Pepper

3 Tablespoons Organic Unrefined Sunflower Oil

Mix ingredients (except oil) in a bowl. Form 6 flat patties. Heat oil in pan over medium-high heat. Add patties and cook until golden brown on each side. Serve alone or as a burger with lettuce and tomato and other sandwich item favorites. Makes 6 burgers.

Awesome Pita Pockets

2 large Avocados, peeled, pitted and cut in thin slices

2 Organic Medium Red or Green Bell Pepper, cut lengthwise strips

2 Portabella Mushrooms, cut into thick slices

1 large Organic Red Onion, chopped

2 Tablespoons Balsamic Vinegar

3 Tablespoons Organic Unrefined Olive Oil

1 cup Organic Sunflower Sprouts

1 cup Vegan Mozzarella Cheese (*Follow Your Heart* brand), grated

8 Organic Pita Pocket Bread halves (4 Pita Pockets cut in half)

1 teaspoon Himalayan Pink Salt

1 tablespoon Crushed Black Pepper

In measuring cup, mix olive oil, balsamic vinegar, Himalayan salt, and pepper together. Place each ingredient to fill pita half and then drizzle olive oil/balsamic mixture. Warm pita halves in oven at 300° F for 3-4 minutes before adding ingredients. Serves 4.

Variations: Drizzle one of your favorite dressings into pita.

Tempeh Burger

1 package Five Grain Organic Tempeh, cut in half lengthwise

2 Tablespoons Nama Shoyu Soy Sauce

1½ teaspoons Ground Black Pepper

1 clove Crushed Organic Garlic

½ teaspoon Organic Cayenne Pepper Powder

½ medium Organic Tomato, sliced

½ Organic Red Onion, cut into slices

¼ cup Organic Unrefined Sunflower Oil

½ teaspoon Himalayan Pink Salt

2 Organic Whole Wheat Grain Buns

2 Tablespoons Vegan Mayonnaise (*Follow Your Heart* brand)

2 Tablespoons Organic Mustard

1 cup Sunflower or Alfalfa Sprouts

In small mixing bowl, combine oil, garlic, cayenne pepper, Nama Shoyu, salt, and pepper and mix well. In large frying pan, heat the oil mixture from bowl over medium heat. When oil is hot, add tempeh squares and cook each side until golden brown, approx. 5 minutes each side. Assemble each sandwich with vegan mayo, mustard, tomato, onion slices and sprouts, add cooked tempeh square and ENJOY!

Makes 2 sandwiches.

Variation: 1 Avocado sliced into strips added to sandwich.

Sausage Cheddar Melt (Healthy comfort food and tastes great)

1 package Gimme Lean Sausage (*Lightlife* brand)

1 Avocado, pitted and sliced

1 Organic Tomato, sliced

6 pack of Whole Grain English Muffins

2 Tablespoons Veganaise Mayo (*Follow Your Heart* brand)

1 pack Vegan Cheddar Cheese (*Follow Your Heart* brand), cut 6 slices

3 Tablespoons Organic Sunflower Oil

Heat Oil in medium fry pan on medium heat. Make 6 patties of Gimme Lean. Place patties into hot oil allow to brown each side, approx. 5 minutes per side. Place sliced cheese on browned side of sausages, cover with lid and allow cheese to melt over medium heat, 3-4 minutes. Toast English muffins. Assemble sandwich with cooked sausage/cheddar, avocado, vegan mayo, tomato, salt and pepper.

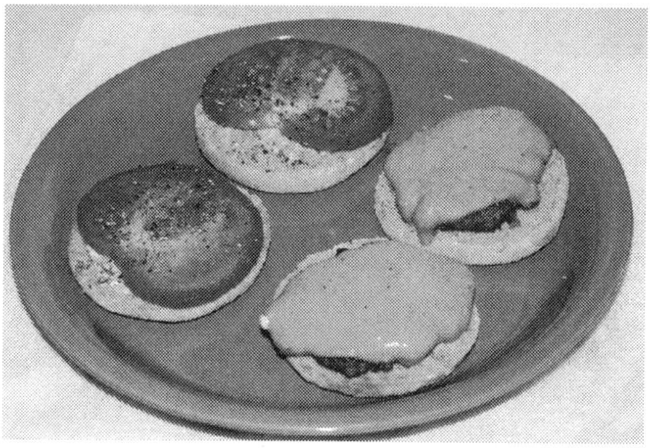

Meat-Less Meat Sandwich

4 slices Organic Whole Grain Bread

8 Tofurky Slices (your choice of flavored tofurky)

½ medium Organic Tomato, sliced

½ Organic Red Onion, cut into slices

½ teaspoon Himalayan Pink Salt

½ teaspoon Crushed Black Pepper

4 Large Leafs of Organic Green Lettuce

2 Tablespoons Vegan Mayonnaise (*Follow Your Heart* brand)

2 Tablespoons Organic Mustard

1 Avocado, peeled and pitted

1 cup Sunflower or Alfalfa Sprouts

Toast slices of bread, then assemble both sandwiches as you would traditional meat sandwich. This sandwich is high in protein, nutrients, taste and NO cholesterol! Makes 2 sandwiches.

Quick Breakfasts

Breakfast is an important meal. You have been fasting all night during sleep, so your body needs some fuel before you start your day. Many studies show eating a healthy breakfast helps balance blood sugars, improves memory function and fewer energy crash episodes later in the day.

<u>Whole Grain Pancakes</u>

1 ¼ cups Organic Whole-Wheat Pastry Flour

½ Tablespoon Organic Raw Agave Nectar

¼ teaspoon ground Cinnamon

1 Tablespoon Baking Powder (use aluminum free)

Pinch Himalayan Pink Salt

2 Eggs equivalence (use egg substitute - see page 86)

1 cup Organic Nut Milk of your choice

Blend together until mixed smooth. Coat Frying pan with sunflower oil and place over medium heat. Make pancakes to desired size. Makes about a dozen. Dress with vegan soy margarine or homemade olive oil butter and maple syrup.

<u>French Toast</u>

6-7 slices of Whole Grain Bread

1 cup Organic Soy Milk, plain or vanilla

¼ cup Organic Whole Wheat Pastry Flour

1 Tablespoon Organic Raw Agave Nectar

1 teaspoon Vanilla

½ teaspoon ground Cinnamon

¼ cup Organic Unrefined Sunflower Oil

Blend ingredients together (except bread and oil) until smooth. Pour some liquid onto large plate and soak bread slices, not too soggy. In large fry pan, heat oil over medium heat and cook soaked bread slices until golden brown, about 3 minutes. Flip with spatula and cook other side of bread. Serve with maple syrup.

Quick Power Cereal

¼ cup Raw Organic Sunflower Seeds, soaked overnight

¼ cup Organic Raw Almonds, soaked overnight

1 cup Organic "Nut" Milk of your choice

1 cup Fresh Organic Fruit

Warm nut milk slightly then pour over cereal and fruit. (Be creative, use strawberries, mango, raspberries, banana). Serves 3-4.

Authentic Oatmeal

Old school, like real old school, perhaps even before fire, but very good for you.

2 cups Organic Raw Oats, soaked 24 hours

1 Organic Apple, unpeeled and chopped

2 Tablespoons Maple Syrup

1 teaspoon Cinnamon

Pinch Himalayan Pink Salt

½ teaspoon Vanilla Extract

1 cup Organic Soy Milk

Raw Oats need to be soaked 24 hours in fresh water. Rinse in fresh water and store in airtight container. They are very good and nutritious. You will love the boost you get from raw oatmeal.

Blend ingredients together, except nut milk until smooth. Warm soy milk and pour over serving of oatmeal. Serves 3-4.

Raisin-Berry Bran Cereal

1 large Bowl of Organic Raisin Bran

1 ½ cups Organic Vanilla Soymilk

½ cup Organic Raspberries or Strawberries

½ cup Organic Blueberries

A great, quick breakfast and the additional berries add antioxidants and spices up the ordinary, boring raisin bran. ☺

Black Pepper Grits

1 cup Organic Corn Grits

3 cups Filtered Water

Pinch Himalayan Pink Salt

4 Tablespoons Crushed Black Pepper

1 teaspoon Organic Unrefined Olive Oil

Bring water to a boil, add corn grits and salt, reduce heat and cook slowly for about five minutes. Remove from heat, cover, and let stand for 2-3 minutes. Stir in 1 teaspoon olive oil and black pepper. Serve with two pieces of whole grain toast with avocado spread, salt, and pepper. Serving size: 1 cup. Serves 4.

Derek's Tofu Scramble

2 (14 oz) Organic Firm Tofu, cubed

3 Organic Green Onions, chopped

4 Organic Roma Tomatoes, chopped

1 package Seitan, chopped (*Whitewave* or *Sweet Earth* brand)

1 cup Organic Broccoli, chopped

1 cup Organic Cauliflower, chopped

¼ cup Bragg's Liquid Aminos

2 Organic Garlic Cloves, crushed

1 Tablespoon Turmeric Powder (Turmeric gives yellow color similar to scrambled eggs and added health benefits.)

In large frying pan, heat ¾ cup sunflower oil with ¼ cup Bragg's Liquid Aminos and crushed garlic cloves, and mix well. Add Seitan, cubed tofu and turmeric. Mash tofu into small parts, simmer for 8-10 minutes over medium heat. Add remaining veggie ingredients and cook 2-3 minutes longer. Serves 4-6.

*For a hearty meal, combine Black Pepper Grits to Derek's Tofu Scramble and allow to stand covered for 5-10 minutes, serve with whole grain toast.

Breakfast Burritos:

A lack of time is often why healthy meals are skipped. So for a great on the go breakfast, make Derek's Tofu Scramble, then simply wrap the scramble into a few extra-large tortillas. Any leftovers can be an awesome lunch to help power you through the day.

Snacks

Most all of the recipes in **The 16/21 Solution** can be used as a snack between meals, after school or work. Here are some other great snacks to replace the usual junk food between meals.

- **Primal Strips:** A variety of flavors, similar to jerky but meat-free and wonderful sources of protein. Found at natural food stores and made from soy and seitan, they make a great snack. You won't believe how good these taste until you try them. The texture is satisfying and cholesterol free.
- **Organic Raw Food Bars:** Excellent source of energy, great tasting and far better than the usual protein/energy bars that are over-processed. These bars have no refined sugars, no trans-fats/hydrogenated oils. No artificial additives, colors or preservatives. No Dairy or soy products. I like *Organic Food Bars, Raw Revolution Bars, Pure Bars, Smart Monkey Bars,* and *18 Rabbit Bars.*
- **Flaxseed Crackers:** Dehydrated flaxseed crackers make a great snack alternative to chips. Eat with salsa, guacamole, or meat substitute items. *Matter of Flax* makes delicious crisps.
- **Organic Fruit:** A great way of getting more nutrients and water into your system. Don't forget to eat plenty of fruit each day.
- **Veggies:** Organic veggies as a snack are great treats that are good for you. Make some quick spreads from my recipes to dip or eat alone. Veggies and are high in fiber and anti-oxidants.
- **John's Trail Mix:** Make your own trail mix. A great friend of mine makes a killer mix of raw cashews, walnuts, almonds and raisins. Place all of the goodies into a zip-lock bag and snack on throughout the day. Makes for a good nutritional snack and curbs junk cravings.
- **Smoothies:** Make one of the smoothies listed in the recipes for a great snack. Try to avoid using the protein powders sold at stores. You don't really need them.

Initially, your taste buds may be in shock when you start snacking on healthier items. Remember the conventional snacks you have been eating most of your life are full of toxic chemicals and flavor enhancers to get you "hooked" on the product and leave you feeling like crud after indulging. It's funny, if you ever had a bad hang over, you never wonder where it came from. The same is true of why you don't feel well due to unhealthy snacks. Under-estimating how much snacks influence your health can be deadly. You will find eating healthier snacks is fulfilling and the physical health benefits show up quickly.

Coconuts: The water and meat they contain are highly nutritious, very tasty, and very versatile. Use coconuts for smoothies, entrees and desserts. You can master coconut opening in no time.

Coconut Opening Lesson:

Using a cleaver, whack downward onto the top of immature (young) coconut to break open, then insert cleaver to wedge open to pour the the coconut water into bowl or blender. Once empty of the water, cut coconut open further until you create a "flip top." Spoon out fresh meat. Add it to the coconut water to blend or set aside for other uses. Raw coconut is one of the most nutritious and healthy items nature has made. for us. This coconut "whacking" sounds difficult at first, but is quite easy after you whack a couple. Do NOT hit your stabilizing hand!!

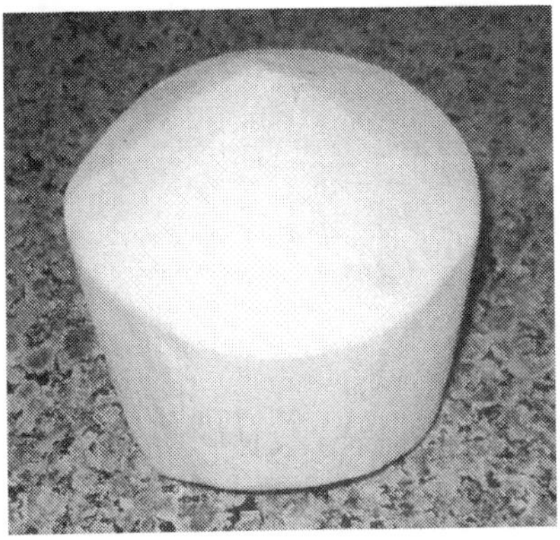

Immature (young) Coconut

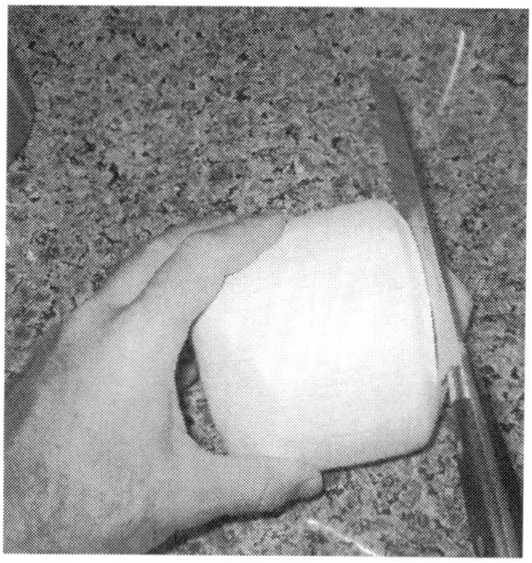

Whack downward with cleaver onto top ¼ of coconut (Caution: Move hand out of the way before hitting downward.)

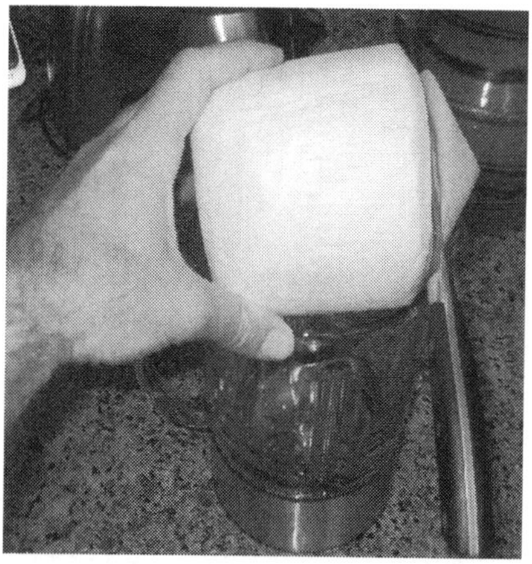

Use Cleaver to pry open coconut to drain the water into blender.

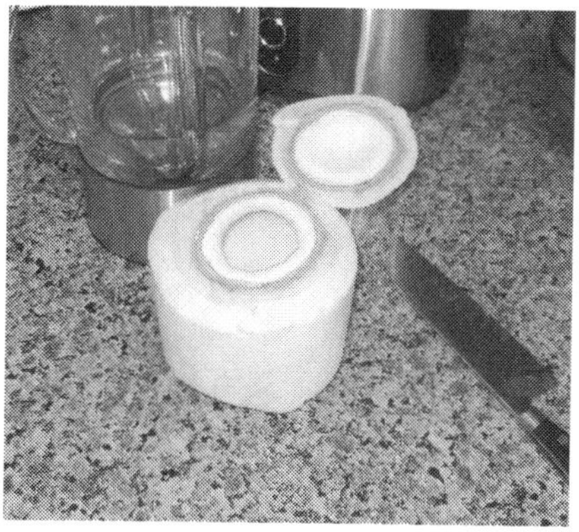

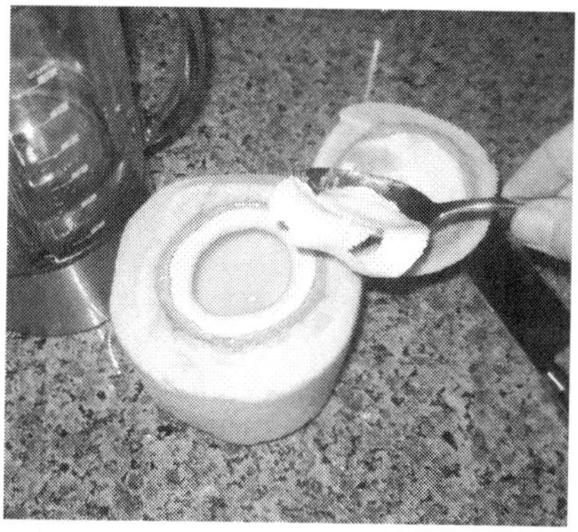

After drained, continue cutting the top of coconut open, make a "flip top" to the coconut to spoon out meat.

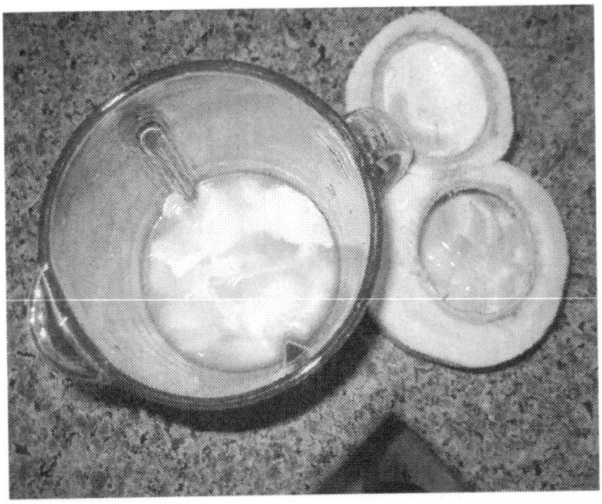

Coconut meat that has been scraped out of coconut and placed into blender.

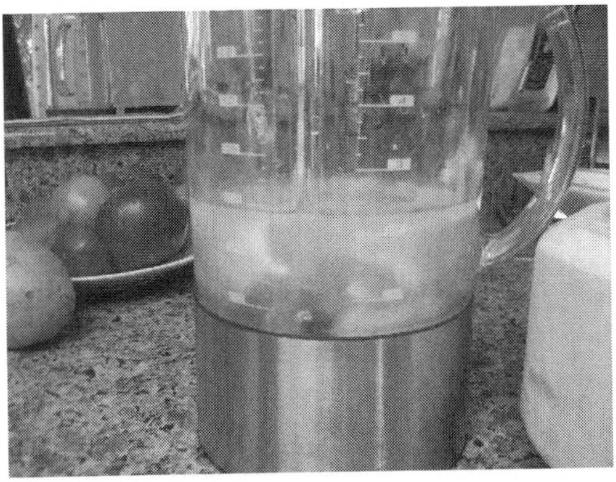

On average, 1 immature coconut yields approx. 2 cups coconut water and 1 cup coconut meat.

Blend well. For some smoothie recipes, I use only the water and save the meat for later use.

Recipe Substitute:

If fresh immature coconut is unavailable, you can substitute organic canned coconut milk on a 1-to-1 ratio. (i.e., 1 cup to 1 cup)

Desserts

Desserts do not have to be a no-no. I think everyone loves a great dessert and these desserts are designed to taste great and provide you with added nutrients. Many desserts we eat are not good for our health, create inflammation, and make us tired—and that's just wrong, but not anymore. ☺

Coconut Chocolate Pudding

2 cups Coconut Meat

1 cup Coconut Water

½ cup Maple Syrup

¼ cup Organic Raw Agave Nectar

½ cup Cacao or Cocoa Powder

Pinch of Himalayan Pink Salt

1 Tablespoon Vanilla Extract

Blend until smooth.

Coconut Milk

2 Immature Coconuts, which should yield:

1.5 to 2 cups Raw Coconut Meat &

4 cups Coconut Water

Place in blender and blend until smooth. Makes 2 cups.

Banana Nog

1 cup Organic Almonds, soaked overnight

3 cups Filtered Water

1 Tablespoon Vanilla Extract

2 Tablespoons Organic Raw Agave Nectar

3 ripe Organic Bananas

1 teaspoon Nutmeg

Place in blender and blend until smooth.

Blow Your Mind Key Lime Pie

½ cup Organic Lime Juice (about 2-3 limes)

1 large Avocado, peeled and pitted

¼ cup Organic Coconut Milk (canned is fine)

½ cup Organic Raw Agave Nectar

¾ teaspoon Vanilla

Pinch of Himalayan Pink Salt

½ cup Coconut Butter (also known as Coconut Oil)

2 Tablespoons Lecithin Granules

Place all filling ingredients (except coconut butter and lecithin) into a food processor or blender. Blend until smooth. Add lecithin and coconut butter and continue blending until creamy smooth. Pour into one of the RAW pie crusts of your choice and chill for an hour or so.

This is a highly nutritious raw pie! ☺

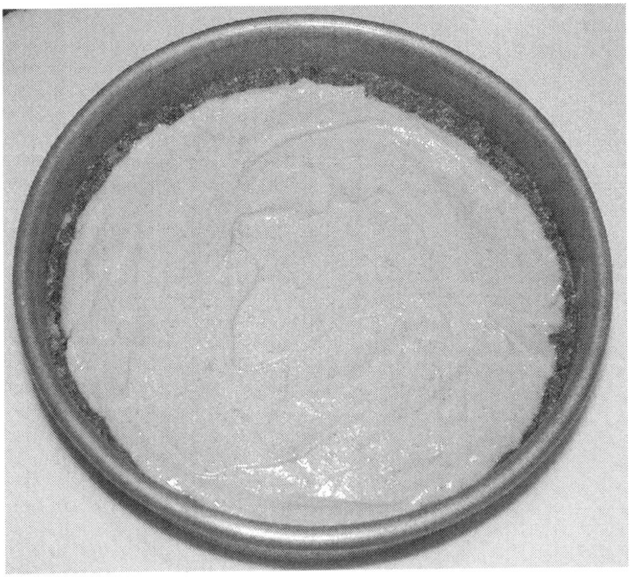

Key Lime Pie

Pumpkin Pie

20 oz Organic Silken Tofu, drained

1 (9-inch) pie crust (*Wholly Wholesome Brand* is low-fat and cholesterol free in the frozen section.)

1 (16 oz) can of Organic Pumpkin

¾ cup of Raw Sugar

¼ teaspoon Himalayan Pink Salt

1 teaspoon Cinnamon

½ teaspoon Ginger Powder

¼ teaspoon Allspice Powder

½ teaspoon Nutmeg Powder

Preheat oven to 375° F. Blend all ingredients in food processor or blender until smooth and creamy. Pour into crust and bake about and hour, or until toothpick inserted into center comes out nearly clean. Allow to cool and chill in fridge if desired. Enjoy!

Healthy Raw Pie Crusts

The frozen pie crusts found at *Whole Foods* and other natural food markets are good, but there is nothing better than making a nutritious homemade pie that is quick and easy, including the crust. Try these RAW Pie crusts for the base of any pies you crave, and remember these are high in nutrients and awesome. ☺

<u>Walnut Crust</u>

1 ½ cup Raw Walnuts, soaked overnight

½ cup Pitted Dates, chopped

2 teaspoons Vanilla Extract

1 teaspoon Ground Cinnamon

Pinch of Himalayan Pink Salt

Place ingredients in food processor, and with S blade, process until dough-like. Press into 9-inch pan.

<u>Almond Crust</u>

1 ½ cups Raw Organic Almonds, soaked overnight

1 teaspoon Vanilla Extract

½ cup Pitted Dates, chopped

1 teaspoon Ground Cinnamon

Pinch of Himalayan Pink Salt

Place ingredients in food processor, and with S blade, process until dough-like. Press into 9-inch pan.

<u>Hawaiian Crust</u>

1 ½ cups Raw Macadamia Nuts

1 cup Dry Shredded Unsweetened Coconut

2 Ripe Organic Bananas

Pinch of Himalayan Pink Salt

Place ingredients in food processor, and with S blade, process until dough-like. Press into 9-inch pan.

Healthy Pie Fillings

Once again, simple, great tasting and good for you.

Violets' Blueberry

4 cups Fresh or Frozen Blueberries

2 Tablespoons Organic Raw Agave Nectar

Blend ingredients in blender well. Pour in your preferred crust. Chill for an hour or more.

Variations: Use Strawberries, Blackberries or Cherries

Apple Pie

4 Organic Apples, peeled and sliced

½ cup Pitted Dates, chopped

1 Tablespoon Organic Lemon Juice

1 teaspoon Ground Cinnamon

¼ cup Organic Raw Agave Nectar

1 cup Filtered Water

Place Ingredients in Blender and blend well. Use a little water to thin for filling texture. Pour into favorite crust. Chill for an hour or more.

Other Awesome Goodies

Here are a few more goodies that will amaze the kids or other non-believers that real food tastes great.

Raw Chocolate Chip Cookies

1 cup Raw Almonds, soaked overnight

1 cup Raw Macadamia Nuts (not soaked)

1 cup Pitted Dates

½ teaspoon Vanilla Extract

1 cup Organic Vegan Chocolate Chips

Pinch of Himalayan Pink Salt

Place all ingredients (except chocolate chips) into food processor. Process until dough-like, but do not over process. Add chocolate chips to mixture, just enough to blend all together. Scoop about 1 tablespoon size into hand and place flatten dough onto a large plate. Chill for 1 hour or more. Makes about 24 cookies.

Chocolate Macaroons

3 cups Dry Shredded Unsweetened Coconut

1 cup Organic Cacao Powder

1 cup Maple Syrup

1/3 cup Coconut Butter/Oil

1 Tablespoon Vanilla Extract

Pinch of Himalayan Pink Salt

Mix ingredients together in large bowl. Use mixer if you prefer. Use a tablespoon to make desired size cookie. Place on cookie sheet at 375° F for 10-12 minutes or until light golden brown.

Coconut Pudding

2 cups Organic Cashews, soaked overnight

1 ½ cup Organic Almond Milk, unsweetened

¼ cup Pitted Dates, chopped

1 cup Dry Shredded Unsweetened Coconut

Blend all ingredients together. You may eat it right away or chill in the fridge. You can also substitute the ¼ cup pitted dates for maple syrup, raw agave nectar, or honey at the same quantity ratio.

Choco-Nut Pudding

1 cup Organic Cashews, soaked overnight

1 cup Organic Almonds, soaked overnight

¼ cup Maple Syrup

1 cup Dry Shredded Unsweetened Coconut

1 Organic Banana

2 cups Organic Vanilla Almond Milk

3 Tablespoons Organic Cacao Powder

Blend all ingredients together. Eat it right away or chill in fridge.

Chocolate Chip Pecan Raw Ice Cream

4 cups Filtered Water

2 cups Organic Pecans

¾ cup Pitted Dates, chopped

1 teaspoon Organic Raw Agave Nectar

1 teaspoon Vanilla Extract

1 cup Organic Dairy Free Dark Chocolate Chips

Blend all ingredients (except chocolate chips) into blender and blend on high to mix well, about 2 minutes. Add chocolate chips and stir. Allow to cool in fridge for 30 minutes, then place in freezer.

This raw ice cream will have a little grainy texture due to the ingredients. This is normal. It tastes great, has a lot of nutrients, and no cholesterol.

Coconut Chocolate Dream Stacks

½ cup Organic Cacao Powder

2 cups Dry Unsweetened Coconut, shredded

½ cup Organic Coconut Oil (aka; coconut butter)

¼ cup Organic Agave Nectar

Mix all ingredients well and use teaspoon to make rounded haystack type balls. Use wax paper on baking sheet or a plate and freeze for at least 1 hour.

CHAPTER 9

Conceptual Approach to Healthier Eating

"Healthy eating" has become a big industry and strategic marketing is used daily in the media. This creative marketing is designed to capture your mind-set and at times contains misleading phrases so you think you are making healthier choices. Remember, your body works better utilizing the foods I have outlined in this book. The following are marketing campaign examples you should be aware of.

Organic Meats:

Organic meats are now advertised and sold as a healthy option for people wanting to reduce their exposure to hormones and chemical toxins. The U.S. Department of Agriculture (USDA) states that animals raised in an organic operation must be fed organic feed, given access to the outdoors, and receive no antibiotics or growth hormones. However, while toxin levels may be less in the animal, switching to organic meat does nothing to decrease the risk of the diseases that remain the top killers of Americans. Cholesterol, animal fat, and animal protein are the major culprits in meat that are associated with higher risks of heart disease, diabetes, obesity, hypertension and some cancers. Animal products, however they are produced, increase the risk of many diseases.

Milk Does the Body Good?:

Significant research suggests dairy milk and dairy products are not good for your health. The dairy industry is a very large business and backed by many government programs and media hype. But to put it in simple terms, we humans are the only species that drinks another species breast milk, and we do it way past the weaning stage. Grown cows do not drink milk! Cow's milk is designed by nature to take an

80 pound newborn calf to an 800 pound animal within the first year of life. Not ideal for human consumption.

Meat and Milk for Strong Bones?:

Osteoporosis is a big health concern, especially for females. Calcium supplements are sold by the tons each year, but the problem still exists. The lack of calcium intake is not the problem. Calcium loss is. Americans have a high incident of osteoporosis but are told to consume animal parts and fluids for better health. However, studies show that animal proteins tend to leach calcium from the bones, leading to calcium loss. Animal proteins are high in sulfur-containing amino acids, especially cysteine and methionine. Sulfur is converted to sulfate, which tends to acidify the blood. During the process of neutralizing this acid, calcium for your bones is released into the bloodstream and then filters through the kidneys into the urine. It is a dietary induced problem, not a mystery illness. Meats and eggs contain 2-5 times more of these amino acids than plant based foods.

Top Killers of Americans ages 55-75:

All linked to **poor diet**. (World Health Organization Stats.)

1. **Heart attack, diabetes and stroke** **52% of all deaths**
2. **All cancers** **38% of all deaths**

I am amazed the promotion of food products that have a direct link to increasing the risk of disease continue to be marketed as "good for you." It actually makes me mad this blatant misinformation is allowed to occur, especially to children, whose lives are just beginning and good nutrition is essential. We live in a free country and are allowed to choose what we want to eat and drink, but unhealthy items should not be propagated as good for you. I have more respect for soft drink makers. They never claim their products do the body good, yet people choose to consume the products, knowing it's junk food. I encourage you to continue to educate yourself for better health. I realize there is a lot of information out there and a lot of it is marketing BS. If you keep in mind that you are built to consume plant-based whole foods for the majority of your dietary intake, then you will do just fine. See the links in Chapter 11 for more quality reading material. Don't get caught up in big business marketing.

Eating Out and Travel:

Eating out locally or while traveling can sometimes be a challenge when eating healthier. However, it can now be a fun adventure. Eating healthier on excursion enhances your travels by providing you more mental clarity and energy. Eating strategy: When you go to a restaurant, it is important to study the menu. Most higher-end restaurants are usually happy to accommodate your healthier eating requests. The typical greasy spoon may be more difficult.

While reading the menu, look at all the ingredients listed in the appetizers, salads and entrees. You can actually build your own meal within the menu you are reading. For example, a salad item will usually contain several vegetables in its creation. Same holds true with the entrées. Many entrées will contain mushrooms, vegetables, rice and pastas. Look to design an appetizer or entrée for yourself that contains a lot of nutrient-rich components. Then tell the wait staff what you want to accomplish. Ask your waiter what fresh vegetables are on hand for that particular day. At many restaurants, I have experienced, upon hearing my questions and ideas, the chef has come out to ask me more elaborate questions. I have found that chef's, by nature, are very creative people and many times your request is an exciting challenge to them. Often times they have to prepare set menus day after day, which bores them to tears. So, they are usually inspired to impress you.

Most menus will be stocked with many wonderful food items you can arrange to your liking and still be healthy. It gets easier, the more familiar you become with working with real foods. Try to look for organic vegetarian and raw cuisine restaurants as first choice. (No, not raw like sushi.) Finding wonderful places to eat healthy on the road is a lot fun. It brings a sense of adventure and usually takes you off the beaten path. I find that enjoyable and enriching. Check the websites I have listed in Chapter 11; (pp 153-155) for a few spots to eat in various places you may be travelling.

CHAPTER 10

Health Tips for the New You

Exercise:

Yes, exercise is important. It helps discharge stress and keeps your metabolism going. 20 minutes a day doing some sort of movement is sufficient. If you work out for longer periods of time, great, but if you do not work out at all, it is probably because you do not like it. It is unlikely you are going to start exercising an hour or more everyday when you don't like it to begin with. Therefore, be realistic. Don't think of exercise as a chore or working out if you have negative thoughts toward exercise. Think of it as going and doing something fun. Try walking. Walk with intention of getting somewhere. For instance, if you are walking with your mate or a friend and you can still carry on a conversation while on the walk, that is a good rate. Walk long enough to sweat a little. If you can walk 20 minutes per day, you will see good results.

My **16/21 Diet Solution** dietary changes are highly valuable to your overall system and you will probably find that you do not need to exercise 2 hours or more a day to experience good results. As a sports injury specialist, I caution you to start slow. I am not an advocate of hitting the weights hard or "jogging" to start out. Give yourself appropriate time to acclimate to more movement. You will stimulate some muscles that have not seen action for a long time and an injury will only set you back. **Go slow**, but do something easy for at least 20 minutes each day. Even if your do 10 minutes twice daily.

Exercises I do recommend in the beginning phase: Yoga, pilates, walking/hiking, treadmill, elliptical, stationary bike, light weights, and swimming. You don't have to "technically" swim if you are not a good swimmer. Going into the deep end of the pool and treading water, running in place and getting general movements of your arms and legs is very beneficial, as water is easy on your joints. However, **if you cannot swim, do not use the deep end of the pool.** The bottom line is: **Do something**, and do something **you enjoy**.

Healthy Living Ideas:

Daily tips:

1. Drink a cup of water upon arising. Water is essential to life and this will help get your body going to start the day.
2. Do a little whole-body stretching. Nothing fancy, just stand and stretch your body out. Have you ever observed a cat or a dog right after they wake up? The first thing they do is a global stretch of their working parts before dashing off.
3. Eat something for breakfast, at least a piece of fruit or whole grain toast with avocado.

Stress Management:

I believe relieving mental stress is essential for a healthier life. Spend some time on yourself each day, even just 10 minutes to think, dream and conjure up thoughts of well-being, happiness, and things you love. It may sound like a bunch of new age blah-blah, but in reality, we become very busy working in life and we forget to play and dream. I believe that is what we all miss the most from childhood, dreaming and playing, so allow yourself a little room to do this. Continue to learn and allow yourself to seek motivation from within. You are your biggest source of motivation. If it means something to you, **you will do it**. Allow yourself this aspect of personal growth. There are many wonderful books and seminars to attend for personal enrichment. There are many self-help resources out there.

CHAPTER 11

Recommended Reading Material, Web Sites & Great Places to Eat

Books

1. **Becoming Vegan: A Complete Guide to Adopting a Healthy Plant-Based Diet.** By Brenda Davis, RD & Vesanto Melina, MS, RD
2. **A Diet For A New America.** By John Robbins
3. **The Food Revolution.** By John Robbins
4. **Living On Live Foods.** By Alissa Cohen
5. **Ani's Raw Food Kitchen.** By Ani Phyo
6. **Eat To Live.** By Joel Furhman, MD

Web Sites

- www.pcrm.org *Physicians Committee for Responsible Medicine:* professional, accurate source for healthy dietary information.
- www.foodrevolution.org enlightened, informative, everyone should visit this site. We only have one planet to live on.
- www.vegsource.com reputable site with many links to good info.
- www.veganreader.com informative and interesting articles about the vegan related world.
- www.drmcdougall.com A very good site for a lot of information regarding nutritional information. A pioneer in medical nutrition.

Restaurants from All-Over

My goal is to list quality restaurants for you to visit that can provide you with good meals that are healthy and align with **The 16/21 Diet Solution.**

West Coast and Beyond

- **Café Gratitude:** Probably one of the best restaurants in the world. San Francisco-based, 10 locations. www.cafegratitude.com
- **Alive Vegetarian Cuisine:** San Francisco, CA. www.aliveveggie.com
- **Greens:** Very good organic restaurant. Fort Mason Center, San Francisco, CA. www.greensrestaurant.com
- **Happy Bamboo:** San Jose, CA. 408-694-0740 www.happybamboo.com
- **Juliano's Raw:** Raw Cuisine. Southern CA: Santa Monica. www.planetraw.com
- **118 Degrees: Raw Cuisine:** Very good. Costa Mesa, CA www.shop118degrees.com/index.html
- **Good to Go:** Huntington Beach, CA. www.goodtogorestaurants.com/
- **Go Raw Café:** Tasty Raw cuisine, Las Vegas, NV, 2 locations. www.gorawcafe.com

East Coast

- **Blossom:** Organic, Vegan and Wonderful. New York, NY. www.blossomnyc.com
- **Caravan of Dreams:** Simply awesome. New York, NY. www.caravanofdreams.net
- **Pure Food and Wine:** Gourmet raw cuisine; owners also have successful raw cookbook. New York, NY. www.purefoodandwine.com

Other

www.wholefoodsmarkets.com: most **Whole Foods Markets** have hot food bar/deli operations. Check website for locations.

www.happycow.net: Wonderful website with locations and reviews of vegetarian and health food restaurants worldwide. I have used them for my overseas travels with accuracy.

Cafe San Pedro: Cartagena, Colombia A wonderful restaurant located in Plaza San Pedro, with vegetarian/vegan options.

APPENDIX A

Glossary of Terms

As all the experts are telling you to eat more vegetables, fruits, nuts and grains, which is very good advice, I still find many patients are confused as to what that means. They are still consuming many ingredients that are toxic in pre-made items and do not realize it. Remember, any time something becomes known in the media, it is going to be heavily marketed and not everything sounding good is good. If you need to re-read this book 400 times, please understand that you, as a living being, need to eat real food, which for humans are all-natural, unprocessed, plant-based foods.
Recently, I saw a commercial from a big name soup company that is now using sea salt. Yes, sea salt is better than conventional salt, but the fact they are marketing sea salt in one of their products does not mean their junk in a can is any better. It has become more marketable, but that does not mean it is healthier. I hope you see my point.

Be careful of marketing terms such as:

All-Natural: All-natural, to me is untouched and unprocessed. If it can sit around for months in a package or a bottle, it is not all natural. Mold and mildew is technically all natural too but not good for you.

Less Fat: Less fat than what? Lard? Be careful of percentages. Values can be misleading and over-marketed with subtle white lies.

Zero Grams: Be careful of misleading labels. Measurement units can be misleading as well. The example, 1 gram is 1000 milligrams. It may say 0 grams of trans-fats, but still may contain trans-fats. The package may say 0 grams, but 999 mg is 1 mg short of a gram, therefore it is not a gram and therefore it may be misleading.

Clinical Note:

You may actually feel a little worse at first when you start pumping the body full of nutrients. This is common, normal, and you can usually expect it. It will pass, usually within a week or two. The length of time varies from person to person, depending on your health status when you start improving your diet. Diarrhea, bloating, gas, and energy shifts are common as well. Healing does take time and eating healthy foods will improve your health.

Always consult with your physician if you have any health concerns or questions.

"The Doctor of the future will give no medicine, but will interest his patients in the care of the human frame, in a proper diet, and in the cause and prevention of disease."

~ Thomas Edison

"If anyone wants to save the planet, all they have to do is just stop eating meat. That's the single most important thing you could do. It's staggering when you think about it. Vegetarianism takes care of so many things in one shot: ecology, famine, cruelty."

~ Sir Paul McCartney

"Nothing will benefit human health and increase the chances for survival of life on Earth as much as the evolution to a vegetarian diet."

~ Albert Einstein

APPENDIX B

Company List

Amy's Kitchen
www.amykitchen.com
Organic frozen foods, soups

Arrowhead Mills
800-749-0730
www.hain-celestial.com
Organic flour, nut butters, pastas, and beans

Bob's Red Mill
800-553-2258
www.bobsredmill.com
Organic flours, grains

Bragg
800-446-1990
www.bragg.com
Liquid amino acids

Cascadian Farms
800-869-7105
www.cfarm.com
Organic frozen fruits/veggies

Celestial Seasonings
800-525-0347
www.celestialseasonings.com
Organic Teas

Daiya Co.
www.daiyafoods.com
Non-dairy, soy-free cheese alternative.

Earth's Best Baby Food
www.earthsbest.com
Organic Baby Foods

Eden Foods
800-248-0301
www.edenfoods.com
Organic pastas, beans, nut milks

Fantastic Foods
800-288-1089
www.fantasticfoods.com
Organic ready-made soups, mixes

Field Roast Grain Meat Co.
800-331-9497
www.fieldroast.com
Veggie meats and sausages

Follow Your Heart
www.followyourheart.com
Organic vegan cheeses, mayos

Frontier Herbs
800-729-5422
www.frontiercoop.com
Organic herbs

Garden of Eatin
800-749-0730
www.gardenofeatin.com
Organic snacks, chips

Guiltless Gourmet
www.guiltlessgourmet.com
Organic snacks

Health Valley
800-434-4246
www.Hain-celestial.com
Organic soups, snacks

Imagine Foods
800-333-6339
www.imaginefoods.com
Organic soups

Island Spring
www.islandspring.com
Organic tofu

Soy Delicious
www.turtlemountain.com
Organic soy foods

Lifelight
800-274-6001
www.lifelite.com
Organic tempeh

Little Bear Organic
800-776-1276
www.hain-celestial.com
Organic chili, soups, snacks

Lotus Foods
www.lotusfoods.com
Organic rice, rice cooker

Lundberg Family Farms
www.lundberg.com
Organic rice, snacks

Maranatha
www.worldpantry.com
Organic nut butters

Miso Master
800-334-5804
www.great-eastern-sun.com
Organic miso

Muir Glen
800-832-6345
www.muirglen.com
Organic tomato sauces

Nasoya
800-462-7692
www.nasoya.com
Organic soy sauce (raw)

Natural Value
www.naturalvalue.com
Organic canned and dry foods

Newman's Own
www.newmansownorganics.com
Organic snacks, dressings

Nile Spice
800-333-4628
www.hain-celestial.com
Organic soup cups

Ohsawa
800-475-3663
www.goldminenaturalfood.com
Organic Asian foods

Pacific Foods
www.pacificfoods.com
Organic veg broths, nut milks

Red Star
800-633-8919
www.redstaryeast.com
High-quality yeast for baking

Rising Moon
www.risingmoon.com
Organic frozen pastas, sauces

San-J
800-446-5500
www.san-j.com
Organic soy sauce (wheat-free)

Sorrell Ridge
800-225-0122
www.sorrellridge.com
Organic fruit spreads

Spectrum Naturals
800-995-2705
www.spectrumnaturals.com
Organic unrefined oils

Spice Hunter
800-444-3061
www.spicehuntcr.com
Organic spices

Starlite Cuisine
949-458-1051
www.starlitecuisine.com
Vegetarian frozen items

Steaz Co
215-321-8330
www.steaz.com
Diet drinks w/out chemicals

Thai Kitchen
800-967-8424
www.thaikitchen.com
Soups, sauces

Turtle Island
800-508-8100
www.tofurkey.com
Veggie meats, hot dogs, deli food

Van's
www.vanintl.com
Organic frozen waffles

Westbrae Foods
800-434-4246
www.westbrae.com
Organic beans, pastas, veggies

Yves Veggie Cuisine
www.yvesveggie.com
Meatless bologna, ham, hot dogs

**WholeFood 365,
Whole Kitchen Labels**
www.wholefoods.com
Organic fresh, frozen, dry foods

Wholly Wholesome
Baked Goods
www.whollywholesome.com

18 Rabbits
415-922-6006
www.18rabbits.com
Organic granola, snacks

APPENDIX C

Product Ingredients to Avoid

This is a list of chemicals and additives that you should start looking for in products. Many of these chemicals are used as fillers, flavor enhancers and stabilizers all for the purpose of product shelf life, not for your benefit. Read the label and avoid these if possible.

- acesulfame-K (acesulfame potassium)
- acetylated esters of mono and diglycerides
- ammonium chloride
- **artificial colors**
- **artificial flavors**
- **aspartame (NutraSweet)**
- azodicarbonamide
- benzoates in food
- benzoyl peroxide
- BHA (butylated hydroxyanisole)
- BHT (butylated hydroxytoluene)
- bleached flour
- bromated flour
- brominated vegetable oil (BVO)
- calcium bromate
- calcium disodium EDTA
- calcium peroxide
- calcium propionate
- calcium saccharin
- calcium sorbate
- calcium stearoyl-2-lactylate

- caprocaprylobehenin
- certified colors
- cyclamates
- cysteine (l-cysteine), as an additive for bread products
- DATEM (Diacetyl tartaric and fatty acid esters of mono and diglycerides)
- dimethylpolysiloxane
- dioctyl sodium sulfosuccinate (DSS)
- disodium calcium EDTA
- disodium dihydrogen EDTA
- disodium guanylate
- disodium inosinate
- EDTA
- ethyl vanillin
- ethylene oxide
- ethyoxyquin
- FD & C colors
- **fois gras** (a truly inhumane industry. www.goveg.com/feat/foie/)
- GMP (disodium guanylate)
- hexa-, hepta- and octa-esters of sucrose
- **Hydrogenated Starch Hydrolysate (HSH)**
- IMP (disodium inosinate)
- irradiated foods
- lactylated esters of mono and diglycerides
- methyl silicon
- methylparaben
- micro particularized whey protein derived fat substitute
- **monosodium glutamate (MSG)**
- natamyacin
- nitrates/nitrites
- OLESTRA (Olean)

- **partially-hydrogenated vegetable oil or hydrogenated vegetable oil (trans fats)**
- polydextrose
- potassium benzoate
- potassium bisulfite
- potassium bromate
- potassium metabisulfite
- potassium sorbate
- propionates
- propyl gallate
- propylparaben
- saccharin
- sodium aluminum phosphate
- sodium aluminum sulfate
- sodium benzoate
- sodium bisulfite
- sodium diacetate
- sodium glutamate
- sodium nitrate/nitrite
- sodium propionate
- sodium stearoyl-2-lactylate
- sodium sulfite
- sorbic acid
- sucralose (Splenda)
- sucroglycerides
- sulfites (sulfur dioxide)
- TBHQ (tertiary butyl hydroquinone)
- tetrasodium ED

I realize changing your lifestyle, even the slightest, can be difficult. There are only a small percentage of people that can jump in and make 180-degree changes right away. Therefore, this book is also dedicated to the majority of you. To those of you: many of my patients, some of my own family and some of my dear friends that have found making changes of improving your eating habits difficult. So to you, I give you "Eat Your Ass Off…Literally with The 16/21 Diet Solution." For I will never give up, nor will I quit trying to find a successful way of helping you help yourself.

~ Mark D. Emerson, DC, CCSP

APPENDIX D

Testimonials

"If you are looking for a delicious, yet do-able way to "healthy up" your diet and your life, look no further. Follow Dr. Mark Emerson's 16/21 Diet Solution and watch your unwanted pounds and health problems go down and your energy level go up!"

~ Michael Klaper, MD, Family and Emergency Physician, Author & Nutritional Researcher

"I started seeing Dr. Emerson in 2002 for nutritional and chiropractic care. After receiving care and implementing his nutritional recommendations, I have more energy and I have been able to sustain my energy levels throughout the golf season. I believe my overall health has improved as well."

~ Jim Furyk, PGA Tour Player, 2003 US Open Champion

"Dr. Emerson has brought a wonderful health improvement solution to the real world. For anyone wanting better health, The 16/21 Diet Solution is the perfect answer. The 16/21 Diet Solution can be implemented by anyone with great results. I personally have lost 52 pounds in 5 months using Dr. Emerson's 16/21 Solution and I now recommend it daily in my practice to help my patients."

~ John R. Marian, DC, Doctor of Chiropractic

Dr. Emerson's 16/21 Diet Solution is not a "diet," but rather a brilliant *healthy lifestyle that didn't deprive me of some of my old vices. I soon learned that foods have their own wonderful flavors when you don't douse them with chemical compounds.*

Losing weight was effortless with the major benefit is the meals are easy. I can make delicious meals in minutes with fresh, healthy ingredients, and have leftovers that will make great lunches and snacks!

The totally unexpected plus was that the psoriasis that I have suffered with since my teens, along with the Irritable Bowel Syndrome with which I had been diagnosed, disappeared. I have tested this several times just to know in my own mind that they are diet-related. Every time I added the meats, dairy and chemicals back into my diet, the Psoriasis and I.B. syndrome returned.

This lifestyle is a "no brainer!" You don't have to give up the things you "can't live without," but you readily find that those same things are really not as necessary as you think they are. I "indulge" in things I know are going to cause me discomfort at times, but it just helps to re-enforce that they DO cause discomfort!

His 16/21 Diet Solution is a very realistic, easy to understand, flexible way to lose weight, gain health and realize a whole new world of foods.

~ JG age 52

Index

D

E

F

G

H

S